Fat Dad,
FAT KID

Fat Dad,
FAT KID

One Father and Son's Journey to Take Power Away from the "F-Word"

SHAY BUTLER and GAVIN BUTLER

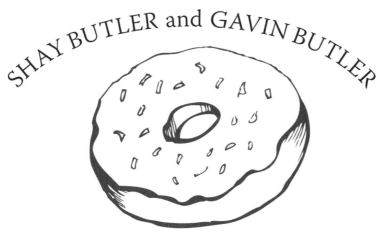

Keywords
PRESS
ATRIA

NEW YORK   LONDON   TORONTO   SYDNEY   NEW DELHI

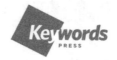

ATRIA PAPERBACK
Imprints of Simon & Schuster, Inc.
1230 Avenue of the Americas
New York, NY 10020

First Keywords Press paperback edition December 2015

Keywords Press and colophon are trademarks of Simon & Schuster, Inc.

For information about special discounts for bulk purchases,
please contact Simon & Schuster Special Sales at 1-866-506-1949 or
business@simonandschuster.com.

The Simon & Schuster Speakers Bureau can bring authors to your live event. For more information or to book an event, contact the Simon & Schuster Speakers Bureau at 1-866-248-3049 or visit our website at www.simonspeakers.com.

Interior design by Dana Sloan

Manufactured in the United States of America

10   9   8   7   6   5   4   3   2   1

Library of Congress Control Number: 2015036008

ISBN 978-1-4767-9231-6
ISBN 978-1-4767-9232-3 (ebook)

Contents

CONTENTS

Foreword

————————————————

by Dave Ramsey

IN 1956, THE GREAT SPEAKER and author Earl Nightingale recorded and released a thirty-minute spoken-word record that literally changed my life. It had already sold millions of copies before I discovered it two decades later. Since I was twelve years old, I've listened to that presentation, *The Strangest Secret*, literally hundreds of times. I could go on and on about the dozens of gems in that talk, but it all boils down to one key point, one central theme, that Nightingale believed was responsible for whatever success or failure any of us ever have in life. That core message is simply this: You become what you think about.

Nightingale believed that success didn't just happen; there is no such thing as stumbling into great success. Instead, he defined success as "the progressive realization of a worthy goal." If you set your mind on something, and if you think about it every day and pour your heart and soul into achieving that goal, you're a success—whether you've hit the goal yet or not.

When I think about that kind of focus and intentionality—what it takes to win in life, money, and business—I can't help but think about my friend Shay Butler. This guy is the walking, talking, *screaming* embodiment of focus. Over the past few years, I've watched Shay set, work toward, and completely crush some incredible goals. Since he lives his life in the public eye through his wildly popular YouTube channel, you've gotten to watch him too. We've all been able to see the intentionality with which he approaches his roles as husband, father, businessman, and even Internet celebrity. You can't help but love this guy.

The first time I met Shay was when he called into my daily radio program, *The Dave Ramsey Show*. On air, I talk to people about personal finance and teach them how to get on a budget, get out of debt, and build wealth. Everyday, people call in to do what we call their debt-free screams. That means they've been working hard over a long period of time to pay off all their debt, except the mortgage, and they're calling the show to tell their story and scream, "WE'RE DEBT FREE!"

One day back in January 2011, I got a call from Shay and Colette in Idaho, who were calling to do their debt-free scream on the air. They told me, and the rest of the country, about their four-year journey to knock out $195,000 of debt! I could tell this guy was focused. We get debt-free calls every day, but talking to a couple who has been so focused for so long on such a huge amount is still pretty amazing. It was obvious that Shay and Colette made an incredible team and that building their marriage and family was a key focus for them.

As the call went on, he told me that he spent the first three years of that process working random jobs as a car salesman and a granite installer, but he had made a career change the fourth year that totally turned his family and his finances upside down. He explained how he had put all of his focus into something he was personally passionate about and gifted at, and as a result had basically quadrupled his income in a year by making YouTube videos with his family!

Later that day, my Twitter account blew up with people congratulating Shay and Colette. I got messages like, "Dave, you just had a rock star call into your show and you didn't even know it!" They were right. I didn't know it at the time, but I had just had met one of the most impressive guys I'll ever meet. We stayed in touch, and we became fast friends.

Not long after that, I joined the rest of the YouTube world in watching Shay tackle his next big goal: weight loss. His business and financial success weren't important if he was putting his health—and therefore his family—at risk by being more than one hundred pounds overweight. As he lost the weight, he and I talked about how we could celebrate hitting his goal, and we decided that we'd run the Nashville Country Music Marathon together. So, about a year later, Shay met me in Nashville and we ran together—for thirteen miles, anyway. I only did the half; Shay ran the full thing!

Over the past few years, I've watched Shay completely smash through every goal he's set his eyes on, from establishing a godly marriage and family to getting out of debt to building a successful business to getting in shape. Now, Shay and his son, Gavin, are focused on a new goal: Making sure health and fitness aren't just a *Shay* thing, but a *family* thing. In *Fat Dad, Fat Kid*, you'll laugh and maybe cry as you always do with Shay, as he and Gavin invite you into their challenges.

In *The Strangest Secret*, Earl Nightingale said, "Every one of us is the sum total of his own thoughts. He is where he is, because that is where he really wants to be, whether he'll admit it or not." You can do or be anything you want if you are intentional, genuine, and focused. And I can't think of a better model for those things than my friend, Shay Butler.

Fat Dad,
FAT KID

Introduction

Does "Fat Dad" Have to Mean "Fat Kid"?

I LOVE BEING A DAD. It's the second most important title I have. Husband is number one, and I'll say more about my amazing wife, Colette, later—I could write a romance novel about that gorgeous woman. But being a good father is an achievement that I'm immensely proud of.

I love my kids so much that it makes me cry. Sitting here right now, thinking about each one of them individually brings tears to my eyes. Colette and I have five amazing children. There's Gavin, who's writing this book with me; my girls, Avia and Emmi; and another two little guys, Brock and Daxton.

The whole reason I started on YouTube was so I could spend more time with my kids. That's another story I'll tell you more about later on, but long story short, I worked all kinds of jobs before I discovered that YouTube could provide for my family and allow me to actually see them on a regular basis. In one of my first ever YouTube videos, I put on one of Colette's unitards and did a pretty damn sexy dance, if I do say so myself. (That dance pretty much sums up why we have five kids—and explains where the Shaytards tag came from.) I didn't know then it would lead me to where I am today.

My kids are my medicine. There are times during my day when I feel overwhelmed or stressed out about a project, or this book deadline, or a comment that I just read on one of our Shaytards vlogs, or any number of things that us humans get stressed out about during a typical day. The only thing that makes me feel better is a good wrestling session with one of my kids. It works without fail every single time. It's like a secret drug that nobody knows about. I'll be sitting at my desk, trying to answer the dump truck's worth of messages that pour into my Gmail every twenty minutes, feeling like crap and on the verge of friggin' out. But then I'll get up from what I'm doing and go hang out with my kids. Now, instead of being a thirty-four-year-old man who has to answer important emails about production budgets, I'm a Velociraptor. As I enter their room with my head bobbing back and forth in a lizardlike motion and my hands clutched in front of my body, mimicking dinosaur claws, I let out a screech that lets my children know a Velociraptor is about to attack them.

What happens next is one of the things I love the very most about children: they don't ask questions about what I'm doing or look at me like I'm ridiculous. They see me and they know I'm a dinosaur, and what do you do when you see a friggin' dinosaur in your room? You scream and run! Then I chase and tickle and bite their necks like any dinosaur would, pretending to rip their spinal cords out through their skins—you know, like any good daddy would. And as they squeal with laughter and giggle uncontrollably, the stress of the world raging inside my head melts away into a puddle of it-doesn't-matter juice.

I love my kids more than I can even explain, and I would never set out to do anything that would harm those who are so precious to me. I want to be a good role model for them and pass on all the lessons I've learned in my life. But there is one thing I'm not proud of, something that I definitely don't want them to follow: I used to be dangerously obese.

Back when I started my ShayLoss channel on YouTube, I weighed in at 281 pounds—and was rapidly closing in on three hundred pounds. I'm five foot nine, so I was almost a square. How did it happen? I was working long hours and then coming home and pulling all-nighters, watching movies from midnight till dawn and fueling those marathon sessions with corn chips and salsa and leftover pizza I scrounged from the fridge. Most days the only exercise I got was hitting buttons on my computer keyboard.

One day I'd had enough—not just of being fat, but of feeling bad. Of not being able to play with my kids without running out of breath. I used to be a vibrant young man who could jump and flip and punch and swim and do all kinds of stuff. But by the age of twenty-nine, I had become a guy who could only upload videos to YouTube. I wanted to feel better. I wanted to be able to ride on a surfboard, glide across a skateboard ramp or ski slope, and do all the exciting, crazy stuff I'd once done. At the time, it didn't seem that long ago that I could do all the things that had given me such a buzz.

I picked up a copy of a book called *Fit for Life* by Harvey and Marilyn Diamond. This is a book that was first published when I was in kindergarten, so it's been around awhile. My parents had it on their bookshelf for my entire life. When I was a nineteen-year-old Morman missionary in Trinidad, I recognized it right away and decided to finally read it. It's all about eating mostly "living" food that has high water content that acts as a kind of natural cleansing agent in your body, especially raw fruits and vegetables. That made a lot of sense to me, so I decided to give it a go to jump-start the process.

Later, after I discovered the Internet, I reached out to Harvey Diamond on MySpace and had a good back-and-forth with him. I told him that his book changed the way I looked at fat, which is totally true—I still rely on its principles to this day. Love it!

Over the next three years, I worked hard, lost over one hundred pounds—documenting the whole process on my ShayLoss channel— and achieved my goal of running a marathon, completing the Los Angeles marathon in March 2012. I'm still dedicated to an active life, and I've kept most of that weight off, but from time to time I slip back into some bad habits and lose my grip on that healthy way of life I know I should be following.

My elder son, Gavin, is eleven now. He and I are molded from the same clay; I think he will have the edge on me height-wise once he's fully grown, but we're both solidly built. We're strong people—if I grab Gavin's leg, I can feel good, solid bone and muscle in there—but it's way too easy for someone with our body type to tip over into being fat. What I want most of all is to pass on to my son the things I've learned about healthy living: the importance of exercising every day and choosing real foods to eat, like delicious, life-filled fruit and vegetables rather than dead-on-the-plate fries and empty-calorie desserts.

But what I fear is that every day, I'm showing Gavin my worst habits: the late-night snacks, the big indulgences, eating until I'm full and then some, the super-size candy at the movies, and getting comfortable on my butt rather than being active and doing the things I love. And I worry that when he sees me falling into those tendencies, he's learning them for himself.

My biggest question is: Does "fat dad" have to lead to "fat kid"?

(I know some of you will hate me using the "F-word" about myself or Gavin. We'll talk about that some more in a little while.)

That's why we're here. Gavin and I have decided to do a father-son healthy living challenge, not only so we can lose weight, but so we can feel our best. We're doing a thirty-day challenge to "go clean," which means no cookies, no candy, no pop, and no ice cream, choosing fresh, nutrient-rich food as often as possible. We're going to drink a gallon of water every day, and we're going to do at least thirty minutes a day of something active, whether it's swimming, or beach soccer, or running, or working out at the gym. Right now, as I write this, it's the beginning of what I hope will be the best summer ever.

Being healthy and finding your most fit body—no matter what the numbers on the scale say—isn't just something you duct-tape onto your life like a makeshift cup holder on the dashboard of your car. No, it has to be a part of your deepest inner life, and the qualities you use to succeed in any area of your life—whether it's your career, or your relationships with your kids, or friendships, or a hobby—are going to be important in reaching your health goals, too. So we're going to be talking a lot about honor, integrity, honesty, and hard work here.

Did I mention the fun though? No one wants to do boring stuff, right? We don't ever want this to feel like work, so it has to be fun. Gavin and I will be shooting hoops, playing soccer on the beach, going for bike rides, and hiking.

Having a buddy to do a challenge with is huge. When I struggle with my weight, it's such a big thing to have my brother Casey, or my good friend Rawn, or my gorgeous wife, Colette, come along to do a workout, or even just eat watermelon with me. Gavin and I figure that if we can do this challenge together, we can motivate each other. This is going to be tough, but we have to talk to each other, we have to take this seriously, and we have to *do* it. We're a team, so if he's having a hard time, he can come talk to me. And if I'm struggling and don't want to exercise, he has to push me.

Gavin and I are keeping a record of our days to show you how things are going, how we feel, which parts are easy, and which ones really suck. We'll also share any ideas we have for making the process easier. Along the way, I'll share parts of my bigger journey, from my midwestern upbringing to some of the bigger health challenges I've faced as an adult.

You'll be hearing from both of us in this book: there are extracts from Gavin's journal here, as well as some actual conversations between Gavin and me as we go through this month of healthy living together.

We're not diet, fitness, or health experts. We just want to show you how we, as regular people, are taking action in our own lives— and taking responsibility for our health and wellness. My greatest hope is that you'll be inspired to take action, too, whether you're a parent who wants to set a good example for your kid, or someone who just wants to make a positive change and feel better.

What would be really cool is if you come along for the ride with us. Do the clean challenge with us so we can all be in this together. I speak from experience when I say: you won't regret it. Gavin is already looking forward to it . . .

I'm excited about this challenge because I want to be healthier so I can play sports better, like soccer and football. But I'm also kind of nervous going into this because I'm lazy and I don't want to do the work. I don't want to exercise and I want to eat junk food.

I've been wanting to lose weight for a while, but I didn't have the urge to get my butt off the couch and work out. But now I'm finally sick and tired of sitting around and not being able to climb a rope or do a handstand. This summer I'm going to be in the best shape of my life. Let's do this.

Day 1

Saying the "F-Word"

THE FIRST THING Gavin and I did for our challenge was weigh in. My view is that your weight is just a number on a scale, and a number on a little device that sits on the bathroom floor doesn't matter nearly as much as how you feel and whether you can do things like dirt bike and Frisbee golf. But it *is* one way to measure progress and changes in your body.

I weighed in at just over two hundred pounds. Aiee, *mamacita*! I want to lose just over twenty pounds. Either I have a lot of muscle or I'm a little bit chubby—the truth is probably somewhere in between. I know what my body would look like at 180. I'll still be solid, but I'll be able to run, climb ropes, do handstands, and jump over deer. At 181, I can't clear a deer. But if I'm 180 pounds, at a full sprint, I can jump over a deer.

Gavin weighed in at 161. That is a great place to start, right here, right now. For him, it isn't about setting a number so much as it's about feeling good and being able to move his body. Once he can jump over a deer he'll know he's where he wants to be.

So we're going to be chasing a lot of deer this summer.

After we finished weighing in, Gavin wrote a list of all the things he wants to do as we get healthier, the things that are maybe hard for him sometimes. Here's his list:

- Boating
- Swimming
- Biking
- Soccer
- Football
- Basketball
- Building a fort
- Skateboarding
- Hiking
- Obstacle courses
- Running
- Dirt biking
- Skiing
- Snowboarding
- Frisbee golf
- Tennis
- Baseball

Man, looking at that list was the kick I needed. I know how it feels not to be able to climb a rope, especially when your little sister can shimmy to the top of the rope, no problem. I know what it's like to want to use your body. You get sick and tired of not being able to do things because your body is too big. Gavin's list pumped me up—it friggin' motivated me. I want to do all those things, too. *Maybe I shouldn't even set a number for myself,* I thought.

But when I watch the old videos I made back when I was really big, I can see what I looked like. What I looked like doesn't even matter; when I look at my old self, I remember how crappy I felt. The heartburn. How much I snored at night. How I would sleep in until one-thirty in the friggin' afternoon. How I could hardly bend over to tie my shoes. How it was as if my belt was the wrong size because it was so tight. I had to stretch out every shirt in my closet before I put it on because they were small on me. I was suffocating myself and felt helpless.

It sucks being like that. I know exactly what it feels like, and I know a lot of people reading this book know exactly what it feels like, too.

On my vlogs, some people write comments like, *I miss the old Shay. The fat, bearded Shay.* Well, the beard comes and goes, but why would they say they miss the fat Shay? Maybe I made them feel okay for carrying extra weight themselves? Because they don't really need to miss me; I'm the same guy in all the ways that matter, but I feel so much better now. I don't feel claustrophobic. I don't feel stuck in a body that won't allow me to do the things I want to do. I can play with my kids without dying from a heart attack. (My maternal grandfather, who was built like me and Gavin, died of one at the age of fifty-three.)

Some people write in to say, *Oh, you weren't fat. Don't say that about yourself.*

Most times, if you say someone's fat, you know it's an insult. In our society, fat is a gross thing. It's important to realize why our society thinks that. Did you know that back in the day, in certain cultures, it was more attractive to be fat? It meant that you were a successful hunter, that you had food to spare. The fatter you were, the better looking you were; the rest of the village would look at you and say, *Man, that fat dude is really making it!* Values have evolved over time, and so have scientific discoveries about health, but that doesn't explain why our society actively looks down on fat people. Most of the time it's not even about a person's health—it's a cosmetic judgment. You can't really talk about someone's health without examining how that person lives his or her life in total.

Here's the other reason fat gets a bad rep: fat is not necessarily bad morally, but it's something that's apparent. You can't hide it if you're fat. You can hide it if you're a jerk. You can hide if you're selfish or a liar. When you eat too much, you can't hide the evidence. It's right there.

Is it worse to be a liar or to be overweight? To me, it's worse to be a liar. I would rather weigh eight hundred pounds than be a liar. Worst of all is a liar calling somebody fat: that makes them cruel.

We need to disarm that word. It's just a word. It doesn't affect me when people use it about me because I used to be fat. I used to make fun of myself. That used to be the basis of my comedy—fat-guy comedy in the tradition of Chris Farley or John Candy. The big men of comedy are some of the greatest.

F-A-T. It's just three letters strung together, and it can mean whatever you want it to mean. To me, fat doesn't matter; it's all about health.

But what about for kids, though? In the schoolyard, it's a word that's often used to hurt others, and that kind of cruelty can't be taken lightly . . .

My dad was asking me, "What do you think about the word 'fat?'" I think if you call someone fat, that's kind of mean. Sometimes other kids have called me fat, and it makes me excited to think about losing weight and showing up at school next year and being really healthy.

One time I was at school and this kid was being mean to this other kid. So I went over there to tell him to back off and leave him alone. And he stood there for a second and then he said, "Eh, um, well at least I'm not fat." I just ignored him and kept playing. But afterward, I thought about it. And even though it doesn't seem like it's that offensive, if you think about it, calling someone fat is kind of offensive.

When I think of the word 'fat,' it's a word that someone tries to use to make you feel bad about yourself. But fat, it's just a word. To some people, it's one of the meanest things you could say. But you just need to ignore it, because you can't let one little three-letter word put you down.

When I think of fat, it doesn't really offend me anymore. My fat, or my blubber, is kind of like my muscle. Being fat makes me big. And being big, to me, means that I'm tough.

Don't be ashamed of being fat. It's kind of dumb when you think about it, getting mad at a three-letter word. Nobody's fat. It's just our stomach is a little bigger than everybody else's.

Another thing is, people call other people fat because they're scared. They're nervous about being made fun of. And I just want to say right now, please don't do that.

This is what I think about the little word "fat."

Day 2

Gavin Goes Sugar-Free

HEALTH IS A PRIVILEGE, and sometimes that fact hits you between the eyes. A couple of years ago, we met a girl known as "the skinniest person in the world." Lizzie Velásquez is a fellow YouTuber and an amazing human being. She also has a rare congenital disease that doesn't allow her to store body fat. She's in her late twenties and she weighs about sixty pounds. She's super skinny and she looks like she has spent time in extreme poverty or a concentration camp. Our family met up with her one evening for the first time.

At first it's startling to see Lizzie in person, so on our way to meet her we explained to the kids that she has a disease that prevents her from gaining weight at all. Gavin was really touched by her because it made him appreciate how lucky he was that his body was healthy. And he was so impressed with Lizzie's positive attitude. Though she doesn't necessarily have control over how others perceive her, she has control over how she perceives herself. That really inspired him, and it also made him realize that *he* had some measure of control. *He* could make a change. That knowledge empowered him to take a step in a healthier direction, so he decided that he would go for a whole year without any refined sugar: no candy, no ice cream, no chocolate, no soda.

GAVIN: Well, it started out when you bet me that I couldn't go that night without a milkshake. So I did that, and then when I met Lizzie, I figured I could do more, so we came up with the bet about going a whole year with no sugar. It became a competitive thing.

SHAY: That's right. I bet you fifty bucks that night, and then you started talking about a whole year. I remember saying to you, "Dude, you're forgetting Halloween." But you didn't ever mess up, did you?

GAVIN: Well no, I wanted that money so I didn't *want* to eat any sugar. After a while, I wasn't craving it. The other thing I noticed when I wasn't eating sugar was, when we went to the dentist, I was the only one who didn't have cavities. I still don't have any.

SHAY: You inspired a lot of people. We announced it on our channels, so everybody watching our vlogs knew about it, and they would try to catch you out. *What is that in his hand? Gavin has candy! Oh, no . . . it's a tennis ball.* I was very proud of you. A lot of people started a similar "sugar fast" because of you. In the comments, people were saying, *If a nine-year-old boy can do it, why can't I do it as an adult?* That's what we need more of in our society: adults making adult decisions, not just doing what feels good.

A lot of adults do what's easy and whatever fulfills their craving in that moment. But in a society that's all about letting yourself do whatever feels good whenever you want, there's something to be said for self-denial. From where I sit, sometimes I worry that it's becoming acceptable to do, feel, and say whatever you want. (That's definitely a big part of Internet culture.) Self-indulgence can be dangerous. There are times when we just have to tell ourselves no to certain things. Refined white sugar is a no-brainer for me, and Gavin and I vow to stay away from it during this challenge.

Before I started saying no to myself, I had close to zero willpower. I've received some criticism about some of the diet choices I've made: eating all raw foods, for one. For my very first weight-loss challenge, I followed a completely raw, plant-based diet, based on the *Fit for Life* program. By doing that, I lost over a hundred pounds and got myself ready to run the Los Angeles marathon. Even so, people thought it was an unhealthy diet. They posted on my comments page, *What about the protein, Shay?* Believe me, that diet was a lot healthier than what I had been doing for many years leading up to it. I used to eat dinner with my family at nine thirty p.m., then when three a.m. rolled around, I'd be watching a movie on Hulu and thinking, *I wonder if there's some leftover pizza in the fridge. . . .* And I would stroll over to that refrigerator, and by golly, there it would be! I'd warm up three slices and drink a liter of Coke while I watched my movie. Do you really think that was a good thing? That raw food diet and what I'm doing now is so much healthier. As for protein, I was eating a lot of nuts and seeds and green leafy vegetables like spinach, which are all packed with protein. Mushrooms are little protein powerhouses, too. You really don't have to eat meat to get all the protein you need to be super strong and healthy. Look at chimpanzees: they don't eat meat, and they're super powerful!

Here's a great rule of thumb for healthy eating, for exercise—for everything you do in life, really. It's based on what I call the "it's better than what you were doing" program. Here's how it works. Just think about one aspect of your daily existence—say, how active you are. If you're like how I used to be, you sit at the computer or in front of the television, then from time to time you get up and walk to the fridge, then you go back to the computer and sit there some more. If you added ten sit-ups or ten pushups or walked around the block once— just once!—it's going to take maybe twenty minutes, tops, and it'll be better than what you were doing before.

Just that incremental change is going to jump-start your progress and give you some momentum. If you do just that one thing for a week, then maybe you'll start walking two blocks around the neighborhood, or running around your one block, or doing ten sit-ups *and* ten push-ups. That's progress. After a while, you might decide to hit the gym or dust off your bike and ride to the park or to your friend's house.

My thing was, I decided to surf. I don't know how to surf, but I tried it one time in LA. It kicked my butt, for sure: I was trying to paddle out to the waves and my arms were burning and the effort was killing me. But it was so much fun, so I bought a wetsuit—there's nothing like that new rubber smell—and a surfboard and had a bunch of good times out there in the waves.

Just this morning, my family and I went down to the beach, and Gavin and I played soccer with the other kids for about an hour. It was such hard work running on the sand, but it felt great and we had a lot of fun. Doing things like that also helps take your mind off the things you're missing, whether you're cutting out Coke or candy or cheeseburgers.

That's the "it's better than what you were doing" program. Do any-thing, so long as it's more—or better—than what you were doing before.

Day 3

Just Call Me Mr. Extreme

Food is delicious. When I'm sad or bored or angry or mad, I eat, so I guess food is kind of like my Kryptonite. Even though I eat when I have these emotions, these past couple of days I've trained myself not to eat all the time. Not only food, but beverages and desserts, too. These past few days, I've only had water and blended juice with fruits and vegetables. With dessert, it's really hard because after dinner you want something sweet—or at least I do. But whenever that happens now, I just have a big glass of water or a banana.

This morning, when I first woke up, I felt like crap. My head was hurting, and I figured that, because it's day three, my body is really starting to notice all the things it's missing. I ate a big slice of watermelon, which helped a little bit. I think I might have been dehydrated—Gavin and I are both struggling to drink enough water. You know we have a goal of drinking a gallon a day, but I don't think either of us has quite managed that yet.

But I can already tell a difference. We went to Rubio's for dinner last night, which is one of our favorite Mexican joints. I love going there. Tacos can be an unhealthy choice when they're piled high with fatty meats and cheeses, and dripping with sour cream, but Rubio's has HealthMex choices that contain less than seven hundred calories for an entire plate of food, with less than 30 percent of those calories from fat. I get a side salad instead of fries and use salsa instead of salad dressing. I also choose corn tortillas for my tacos, which are less caloric than flour tortillas. Normally I would have drunk a ton of Coke with those tacos, but instead I got a bottle of water. I feel like I digested the food in my system a lot faster because I didn't have all that pop. I can't believe we're on day three already—it's crazy how quickly the first few days have gone by.

Whenever I do any sort of health challenge—thirty days of raw foods, or training for a marathon, or this challenge Gavin and I are doing now—people leave critical comments on YouTube. *But Shay, you always take it to the extreme—how about some moderation. Wouldn't that be a better way of making healthy changes in your life?*

It's an excellent question and a very good and valid point. But that's just who I am—the kind of personality I have. In order for me to get excited about something, it has to be big. I love the idea of a challenge of any kind, and something that goes for twenty or thirty days is great because there's a definite end to it. It's not exciting to me to lead a moderate life. Unless there's something ahead of me that's big and outlandish and crazy and difficult, almost to the point where I can't do it, I won't get excited about taking the next step. I just get . . . bored.

Maybe that's a personality flaw of mine, but in order to change, sometimes you have to go hard—at least in the beginning. That's what I want to do for these thirty days. I want to go balls to the wall. Gavin and I are doing a good job, too; we've been playing soccer, going for bike rides, drinking lots of water—we haven't quite been meeting our target of a gallon a day, so we need to tackle that one—eating clean, staying well away from pop and candy and ice cream, which is not easy in the summer, I'm telling you. And I don't believe we'd be achieving all of that if we didn't take a stand and decide to go all out.

I admit that the thirty-day "eating clean" challenge is a little extreme—we're not going to be able to live like this forever. But Gavin and I want to do it for one month so we can say, "We accomplished a hard thing." We set a goal, a measurable, attainable goal, something that forced us to look at a calendar and say, "For the next thirty days, we're going to do this thing." We know it's going to be hard, but we're going to persevere. We're going to get to week two, we're going to go out to eat with our family, we're going to want to cheat, we're going to want to have that day where we can eat anything we want, but we're not going to do it. And then, once we get through these thirty days, we'll know that we can do it. Living without all that extra sugar and with maybe one cheat day a week will be easier from then on out.

"Tomorrow" never comes. You have to set a date. That's why I always like starting something new at the beginning of the month. I'm such a sucker for January 1st: I love that new year, new you kind of vibe, and even though I have failed at multiple resolutions multiple times, I still feel excited about refreshing my life on January 1st because it's a great time to start and draw a line in the sand.

So this month we're going to go hard. We're going to do the hard things, the things we usually procrastinate doing. We're going to take it to the next level.

Most of us live our lives on a linear path: some of us are gradually getting healthier and fitter as we become more health-conscious, and some of us are gradually doing less and eating more. Either way, it's slow going. But if you take one of these hard months and kick your lifestyle into high gear, I believe you can either turn the downhill slide around or boost your improvement up to the next level. I think it's all about pushing yourself and taking those moments to shoot forward, maintain, and then keep going up, little by little. In every aspect of my life, I want to live this month to the fullest, in the way I know I can live.

I'm comfortable, after all. I'm a successful guy. Just before Gavin and I started this challenge, we had the best month ever on Shaytards, coming in at more than 93 million views, so I'm making good money. And sometimes I say to myself, "I'm not struggling to make ends meet, why push it anymore? Why not just relax? Why not just enjoy life?" The answer is because it's not about money, and I know I can do more. When I know that I'm not doing everything that I could, it's like I'm selling myself short. I'm not giving it all that I have.

I know some people don't think that's a healthy or a sustainable way to live. A lot of people want to attack me in the comments—or try to find my weaknesses or what I'm doing wrong, calling me a yo-yo dieter. *Shay lost all this weight. Then he got fat. Then he got lazy. Then he ran a marathon. It's so unhealthy.*

You're right. I have weaknesses. I'm not perfect. I'm the very first person to admit that. I make mistakes all the time, and I am an extremist. That is a thing that I've dealt with my whole life, it's just something that is in me. I am either one hundred thousand percent on or I don't care. That is definitely something that I need to work on.

Here's the thing, though. When people are so anxious to post their comments about my weight-loss videos and try to show how I've messed up or how I've made mistakes, that's not hard. It's pretty obvious. I make a video of my life every day. My entire process of losing over one hundred pounds is right there on YouTube. You can go watch it. I've gained a little bit of that weight back but I haven't gained much more than twenty pounds. I would say to keep around eighty pounds off for three years is pretty good.

I'm not going to stop making these videos just because I say to myself, "I did it again. I got all excited about doing something. I didn't totally do it like I said I was going to do it." I'm going to keep pushing forward. I'm going to keep getting excited about recommitting to my goals. I'm never going to quit, ever.

Day 4

I Love Melons! But I Love
My Wife More

HERE'S ONE THING I need to make clear. I really, really love watermelon. It's like the fruity equivalent of gold to me. It's my savior. If it wasn't for this delicious fruit, I couldn't do this healthy challenge. Every time I feel hungry at night, I cut me up a big, ripe slice of juicy watermelon and eat it. And when I wake up in the morning, the first thing I want is another slice of watermelon. If I were stuck on a deserted island, the one food I would want to have with me would be watermelon. There's nothing like a cold, crisp, freshly cut watermelon on a summer's day while sitting out on the porch in the late afternoon, glistening with sweat after mowing your lawn and turning on the sprinklers, and you can smell that wet, cut-grass smell.

But what I love even more than watermelon is a beautiful woman named Colette who, against all reason, agreed to be my wife. The very first time I saw her I said to my friend, "I'm going to marry her." Which might be kind of creepy, but it worked!

I was raised as an active member of the Church of Jesus Christ of Latter-day Saints, who most people know as "the Mormons." After graduating from high school, I went on a full-time church mission to the West Indies for two years. Most young people in our church go on a mission; it used to be that men had to be nineteen to serve, but a few years back they lowered the age to eighteen for men and nineteen for women. I served in Barbados, Trinidad, and Guyana. When you're on mission you're not permitted to be within one foot of a girl—there's no dating at all—so I was away from all possibility of romance.

Once I got home from my mission, I started to make plans to go to college at Idaho State University in Pocatello. My friend Derek invited me to go with him to see the musical *Anything Goes* because his brother was part of the local community theater group that was performing it. A nineteen-year-old brunette by the name of Colette Crofts was playing the role of Reno Sweeney, a classy nightclub singer on a cruise ship. She came out on stage and straight away I thought, *She is so hot!* She was beautiful—and man, she could *sing*. It was love at first sight. Right away, I checked the program to find out what her name was. Sitting there in the theater, I leaned over to my buddy Derek and whispered to him, "I will marry that girl."

I was captivated, but even so, after the play ended, I was too bashful to join the line of people waiting to meet the cast, so I hung back like a stalker while everyone else in the audience went up and shook hands with the cast and told them how great their performances were. I was too afraid to even talk to this gorgeous woman. Later, I saw her coming out of the philosophy building on campus as I was going in. I remember thinking, *That's the girl from the play! The one I said I was going to marry!* Then I discovered she had a class in the same building as me on Mondays, Wednesdays, and Fridays. Needless to say, I *really* looked forward to that class.

Like a true stalker, I haunted her steps around campus for the next three weeks until I finally got up the courage to ask her to go wakeboarding with me. Totally romantic.

I had never been nervous like that before. Colette thought I was just a naturally shy person, but luckily Derek explained to her that I was actually wild and crazy. (Thanks for that, Derek.) Even more luckily, Colette thought that was okay, so we went wakeboarding at the reservoir with a bunch of friends. I brought my little brother, Logan, with me—my mom made me take him, and I was worried that Logan would say something stupid and embarrass me. But as it turned out, Colette thought it was so sweet that I brought him, so that got me points. I'm sure my cool wakeboarding moves helped, too, not to mention lunch at Subway afterward. (I treat my ladies real nice.)

After that date, I felt just like I thought I would: I was totally in love with the girl. I would have proposed at the end of the first wakeboard wreck, but I felt like that might come across as a little forward. After a lightning-fast two-month engagement, we were married at the Idaho Falls LDS temple on January 3, 2003.

Over a decade and five kids later, I'm just as much in love with that gorgeous brunette as I was when I first saw her up there onstage. Because of our faith, Colette and I believe that we are married not only until death do us part, but that our bond is sealed for eternity. We believe that we live after this life, and that we will remain in this relationship after we die. That means we're an eternal family: our children are sealed with us, and we will always be together.

So what does this have to do with day four of our challenge? Nothing, really. I was just feeling the love today. Or maybe it has everything to do with it, because staying healthy to live longer and have a great life with the family I love so much, and with whom I will be for eternity, is what this is all about.

Day 5

Eat the Friggin' Carrots!

Another question that my dad has asked me is: "Does a cheeseburger really taste better than a cucumber salad?" I thought about it. And I think that a cheeseburger only satisfies our taste buds. But really a salad is better, even though it might not taste as good as a cheeseburger would. It's better for our bodies.

I'm just being honest, but I would probably choose a cheeseburger because it tastes better.

Trust me, guys, I love food. I love cheeseburgers, I love pizza, and I love an ice-cold Coca-Cola Classic on the rocks. You don't know how much I love Coke. Last week I drank a whole two-liter bottle in a day. That's one of the bigger problems I've faced during this challenge: quitting Coke.

Last night I felt like crap. I had the worst headache from caffeine withdrawal, and my body was rebelling against me. These first three to five days have been like the detox period for an alcoholic. My body is addicted to caffeine, so when I don't have it, my body says, *Where's the caffeine? Something is wrong here—give me caffeine!*

If you're giving up caffeine, too, you might find that your muscles ache, you get headaches, and it's hard to concentrate. You might feel tired. But you've just got to get through those first three to five days, and all of that will level off. You'll start to feel better again, and before long you'll feel far better than you did before.

I figure I should explain what I mean about cutting out sugar as part of this health challenge. Our whole extended family came over to our house for Brock's birthday this past weekend, and on the table was broccoli salad with sunflower seeds and some crumbly bacon topping. The recipe calls for a cup of sugar in the dressing. I was eating that broccoli salad and Devri, my wife's sister, said, "I thought you weren't eating sugar."

"Well, we're not being that strict," I told her.

There's some sugar in the foods that we're eating on this challenge: we're eating fruit, which has fructose in it, and dairy foods, which have lactose. We're still getting sugar, but we're cutting out all of that excess sugar that Americans (as well as other Western cultures, too) tend to have too much of: dessert with every meal. Our bodies need sugar to give us energy, fuel our muscles, and keep our brains ticking. What Gavin and I are doing is cutting out processed foods with added refined white sugar, which adds calories to your diet without giving you much else. And not only does it adds empty calories, consuming too much added sugar means our bodies have to go to work processing it instead of doing other important jobs, like protecting us from bugs and viruses.

There are good fats and good sugars out there, people. That's why I hate diets that say you should not eat any fat or any sugar. *Don't eat carrots, they have sugar in them*, people say to me. Shut up! What should I eat instead, suckers and cheeseburgers? Yes, you should eat carrots. Yes, they have sugar in them, but they're good for you: they're low-calorie—a half cup of raw, chopped carrots has just twenty-six calories—and they're packed with fantastic nutrients. Beta-carotene is their big thing: it makes them that funky bright orange color. But more importantly, your body converts it into vitamin A. Not only that, beta-carotene is a mighty antioxidant, so it's good for lowering your risk of heart disease and cancer. So eat the friggin' carrots!

Here I am, getting all worked up about carrots. Let's move on.

I'm going to share with you guys what Gavin and I had for lunch today. I made the most awesome salad. First, I got a mixture of romaine and spinach leaves. The darker the leaves, the more nutrients it has, so I always look out for those dark green leaves instead of light green ones, like iceberg lettuce. I added in tomatoes and cucumbers, then threw in some dried cranberries; sunflower seeds, which are high in protein; and a ton of cashews for protein and crunch. I like something crunchy in a salad; it makes it feel more substantial. Then for dressing I mixed up some extra virgin olive oil, which is beautiful and natural, and some apple cider vinegar—this particular kind of vinegar seems to help with controlling your blood sugar levels, which is pretty cool. Then a little bit of lemon, a little sea salt, and some chopped up garlic. It was a huge bowl of salad, and we ate a whole lot for our lunch, then saved a portion for later on. Just keep eating it throughout the day—that will keep your metabolism going.

Which brings me back to the sugar question. Eating too much processed sugar is not something to be blasé about. All the reports that are coming out now reveal that sugar is a real killer. Eating too much makes our blood sugar spike—that's the feel-good high you get from your morning muffin—then drop down, leaving you in a slump and wanting more. The World Health Organization says that only 5 percent of our daily calories should come from added sugars—so depending on how big you are and whether you're a man or a woman, that's around five to eight teaspoons per day. Teaspoons, not tablespoons or cups or anything else. Trouble is, sugar is tucked away in all sorts of food you wouldn't expect, like bread, pasta sauces, soups, and juice. Soda pop is one of the worst; it's like liquid sugar. It's so easy to chug down a liter, then go for a refill when you're eating out. The companies who sell it know it's full of addictive chemicals—that's what makes it so easy to sell. All the time they're coming up with new ways to make it more appealing, to counter all the research that's coming out. Even if you haven't bought a Coke in five years, you walk into a grocery store and they have a Coke bottle with your name on it, and that's hard to resist. They even have one with "Shay" on it, and I want to buy one because I have the kind of name you never see on key chains at the gas station. So if I see my name on a product, I want to get it. Coke tastes good and it's fun to drink, but it's not good for you.

You just don't realize how sweet these drinks are until you abstain from them for a while. Gavin was saying he noticed that after his year without sugar.

GAVIN: Yeah, we went to a restaurant and I got a root beer and it was super sugary.

SHAY: You forget how syrupy it is. I guess your taste buds changed because they had become desensitized, and all of a sudden you were hit with that sugar. The same is true of salt and fat. If you come back to them after cutting back, their flavors hit you like a brick between the eyes.

When I was training for the St. George Marathon in 2012, I cut out pop and went totally vegan. I was eating all fresh fruits and vegetables, and a ton of nuts, granola, and chia seeds. I was eating thousand-calorie bowls of granola and nuts—I needed a lot of protein because I was running fifteen miles a day. That's probably the healthiest I've ever been, and I felt amazing. It's such a testament to what exercise and good food does, because there were times I felt superhuman. I could run fifteen miles, come home and shower, have my big bowl of granola and a banana, and then I would just work all day long without ever feeling tired.

After I ran that marathon, I decided, *Okay, I deserve some cheat meals now.* That same day, right after I finished the race, Colette went to Wingers and got me a big bacon double cheeseburger with fries and a Coke. It was fun to eat, but I felt like crap afterward. Even when I was chewing it, I could taste that there was too much salt. When you've been eating healthily, your taste buds change and your palate becomes attuned to milder flavors, so when you go back to having all that greasy, sugary food, your body says, *Whoa, whoa, remember what we were doing? We were feeling good. Why are we doing this again?*

Why is that not a signal to us? The first time you eat bad, greasy food after a long break away from it, it doesn't necessarily taste good, and afterward you feel like crap. So why do you think, *I'll try it again?* Your body will get used to you that trash, and it'll get addicted all over again to those chemicals: sugar, salt, and saturated fats. Your body will start wanting that stuff, and then you'll slip back down the path of least resistance.

That's how heart disease has become the number-one killer of people in the world: over time, we slip down these paths of least resistance. You might think that kids would have a harder time than adults giving up things like cookies and candy bars, but it's easier for them because they haven't become addicted over a long period of time, like us grown-ups. As the years pass by, we get into the habit of eating easy, cheap, tasty food because we like the accessibility—and it just tastes good. Those foods give you the instant dopamine stimulation that we're all craving, but there's no nutritional value. The only reason companies make those products is to give the consumer what they want, which is that fast high, that immediate dopamine release. There's sugar and caffeine and salt in abundance in all of these snacks, and people just get into the cycle of eating them. Bob and Lisa are going to work, they're raising their families, and they're stopping at Starbucks every day. First they move from tall to grande to venti beverages, and then after a while Lisa adds whipped cream to her mocha, and Bob adds a chocolate chip muffin to their order. Suddenly, Bob and Lisa are fifty to sixty pounds overweight, they're struggling to breathe after they walk up a flight of stairs, they're feeling bad about how they look, and their doctor is telling them their blood pressure is through the roof.

It just happens—it happened to me.

Day 6

Gumball Addict or Millionaire?

Well, it just gets harder and harder every day. Yesterday we went out for dinner and I was going to get a Sprite but then I remembered I couldn't do that, so I got water. It was tough but I felt good, and I knew I could do it because we were doing it together.

We're at home this afternoon, and as I write this, I can see Emmi and Avia over at the table eating bowls of ice cream. Man, that looks delicious. All right, I'm looking away. I'm looking away. I'm looking—right at those darn bowls of ice cream.

If you eat foods loaded with fat and sugar, your willpower gradually runs out from the time you wake up in the morning. Everyone has a finite amount of willpower, so as you go through the day, being strong and eating good foods, by the time it's eight o'clock at night, you're all out of willpower—you're just sick of the struggle to do the right thing. In the past, when I was letting myself have sugar, I noticed that I'd wake up, eat a healthy breakfast of fruit, exercise, come back, have a protein shake with water and an apple, and have a pretty good lunch of something healthy. It made me feel great. But by the time dinner rolled around at seven, I just wanted to eat something—and by something, I mean *anything*. And I was still ravenous after dinner.

Now that we're doing this challenge, that doesn't happen so much: the swings in energy are less extreme. Even so, it seems harder and harder to make good choices as the day goes on.

The choices you make at midnight are just as important as the ones you make at the breakfast table. We oftentimes don't think about the long-term effects of our small, daily decisions, but they're the things that can lead us to the electric chair or to the White House. Does that sound extreme? Well, it's not! It's the truth, and every day I see it more and more.

After my two years of mission in the West Indies, when I returned home to Idaho, I had never felt more motivated and determined to live the best life I could live. I had just spent twenty-four months helping others overcome the endless struggles that we all encounter, so I was more driven than ever to become the best "me" possible. I felt like

I could accomplish anything—I was twenty-one years old and ready to conquer the world!

A few weeks after I got back, I was shopping at the mall with a friend when I discovered a magical place that would change my life forever. This wonderful place can be found tucked away in your local bookstore. It's a magical treasure trove of truth that has a little placard at the top of the shelf proclaiming itself as the "self-help" aisle.

The self-help section of the bookstore became my sanctuary. I would walk in there and browse through walls of books for hours on end. I love authors like Robert Kiyosaki, Dave Ramsey, Dale Carnegie, Napoleon Hill, Stephen Covey, Zig Ziglar, and Tony Robbins. I was interested in business and success. More than that, I wanted to find the secret to life and live it.

The only problem was, I only had twenty bucks in my wallet. I was a twenty-one-year-old man with a high school diploma, living with his parents and borrowing his mom's cell phone and car. The net worth of all of my earthly possessions was less than one hundred bucks. So you can imagine that spending one-fifth of the contents of my entire bank account on a book with a bald guy with a goatee on the cover was a major sacrifice. On the rare occasions when I could afford to buy one of those books, I made it a rule to read *at least* the first three chapters before handing over my hard-earned cash. I wasn't afraid of being judged for sitting on the floor in the self-help section for thirty minutes, reading as much as I could, even though I got some strange looks from the staff.

Over time, I started to sense a common theme among all of the different authors I was reading. I began to learn that the things you do are more important than anything you say or think. The actions in your life are what make you *you*. I was learning that my habits were the things that made me who I was. Those tiny, daily decisions that most of us don't think are significant are actually the things that bring us to the depths of desperation or raise us up to the glorious heights of elation.

The small things matter. Do you save your extra change in a jar, or rush to the gumball machine to get a wild cherry orb that will be full of delicious flavor for fifty-seven seconds before turning into rubber cement in your mouth? Do you realize that over time, and with compound interest, that saved change could accumulate with other bits of small change and make you a millionaire?

I like the idea of "natural consequences" a lot. In the case of health, it's not so much that if you eat a cupcake, you're going to instantly be in trouble. But the natural consequence over time, if you keep making those same choices, is that you will be less healthy. You won't be able to run around with your kids as much as you'd like. I don't like the feeling that I'm going to get in trouble or be punished. Even as a person who believes in God, I don't believe God gave us commandments to rope us in, or to say, "You have to follow these rules or else." I think they're stepping-stones, given to us to help us.

The greatest thing we have as people is our freedom to choose—what you might call "agency." A lot of people talk about free agency in the sense of not having to answer for their actions to any authority. "I have free agency and I can do whatever I want." But there is no free agency, because every choice you make costs something.

For every action, there is a reaction; that's one of the operating principles of the universe. If you're in science class and you mix two chemicals in the same proportions and under the same conditions, you're going to get the same reaction every time. You can't change that reaction; the universe is in charge of that deal. So when you make a choice, you have to deal with the consequences. Sure, you have the freedom to choose, but there are always consequences to the choices you make.

For Gavin, this is a huge thing to learn right now. Sometimes I think, *Dude, this is your life. I'm your dad, so from the viewpoint of society, it's my job to tell you what to do, but you ultimately have to choose what kind of person you want to be. This is the time for you to be thinking,* This is my life. Who do I want to be? *Don't just do things because Mom and Dad say so, do things because you have a vision of who you want to become. What kind of person are you? And what kind of person do you want to become? Maybe you want to be a hero or a champion. Maybe you want to do something great: be the best soccer player in the world, or inspire people through the things you say and the things you write.*

Sometimes, asking yourself these questions is the only way you can drive yourself on, because motivation is hard to find. It's like what we were saying before about willpower: it's a substance that you can use up and then look high and low to find. Some days it's hard to feel motivated to work out, or to eat a healthy breakfast. Sometimes the only way for me to motivate myself is to ask myself those hard questions: *What am I doing here? Who do I want to be? What kind of person am I?*

There's a saying that the most successful people are the ones who are willing to have the hardest conversations, even with themselves. Our lives are full of problems that we have to overcome every day. We have a headache, or our car battery dies, or someone lets us down.

We are constantly bombarded with stimuli that could erode our motivation and our will to do good things.

Here's the cool thing about agency, though. When it comes to your feelings, you *do* have the power to choose how you feel. You may feel a certain emotion because something made you feel it, but you don't have to keep feeling that way.

Let's say I go to cross the road and some guy is driving by in his truck and I walk out in front of him.

Get the f%$ out of the way!* he screams.

Screw that guy, I might think, and be all pissed off about it. Or I might think, *Oh crap—that was my bad, I did something stupid. But no one got hurt. I'll pay more attention next time.*

Or maybe I'm driving and somebody gets mad at me for cutting them off, and they honk and throw their hands up. I can get mad and be really pissed at them, or I can choose to tell myself, *Chill out, it's not worth it.*

Whether you're eleven years old or fifty-one years old, you can choose how you react to the things that happen to you. When bad things happen, the conversation that happens inside you goes something like this: *My sisters are annoying and now I have to write this essay for school. Why did my teacher give us this essay to write when there are only three days of school left? We should be partying! I'm going to eat some candy now, because food makes me feel good.*

That's what the eleven-year-old might think. If you're the guy who's fifty-one, your thought process might be more along the lines of: *My boss is busting my ass about getting this job done, my car needs new tires, I'm going to spend a half hour in this line at the supermarket. I'm in a bad mood, so I'm going to buy that giant-size bag of potato chips and a case of Keystone Light to make me feel better.* Either way, you want to eat because it feels good, right? But the natural consequence of this kind of attitude is going to make you gain weight. You're going to get fatter.

Eating something like that might make you feel better for a minute, but ultimately it doesn't solve your problems. You still have to write that essay. You still have bratty sisters to deal with. You still have to face up to your boss, or your bills, or the supermarket line. You still have to solve all those problems that you would have to solve anyway, but now you're fatter. You tried to escape the problem by eating, and we all do that. Everybody has a different thing they try to use to help them feel better, whether it's alcohol, smoking, food, gambling— everybody has their own substance or activity that they turn to for a "feel-good" moment. But we have to make wise decisions based on the future instead of what's going to make us feel good right now.

You're in charge. It's your choice. The whole darn shooting match.

Day 7

No More Liquid Sugar

COLETTE LOVES HER CANDY, so she has stashes of candy in the cupboards, way up high or tucked behind the granola. But I know where they are . . .

I'm doing well with it for now, but way back before I first started trying to get healthy, I would sneak those candy stashes out and have a late-night feast. I find Emmi doing it now: she has inherited my sweet tooth and it's a crazy thing. You know that feeling when you eat so much sugar your face gets red and you can feel your heart racing and you say to yourself, *Whoa, I've just eaten about a ton of sugar*? I would eat candy to that point almost every night. Then I'd go to bed, and my body would be saying, *Man, I can't friggin' sleep because I have to get rid of all this crap you just put in me.* And when I'd wake up in the morning, I'd be all groggy and my mouth would feel like someone had come along with a cement mixer full of glue and poured it right in there. My body would be packed with all these chemicals, and it would try every which way to get rid of them.

Last night I wanted that sugar hit again, something sweet before bed, so I ate a big apple, and it felt great. A nice, juicy apple is naturally sweet so it satisfies that craving, but there's also fiber to tell your stomach it's full, and plenty of hydration because your body wants that, too—it just doesn't know how to tell you that. Best of all, if you eat an apple instead of candy, when you wake up in the morning, you won't have a sugar hangover.

Yesterday, Gavin and I bought freshly squeezed juices from Rainbow Acres, which is one of my most favorite places in LA. They have this awesome juice bar where they use all organic fruit and vegetables, so their drinks are packed with vitamins and minerals. I felt so good afterward, I could definitely feel the nutrients surging through my body. Energy, too. When I eat a really good, big, crunchy apple, I can feel it giving me an energy hit. On top of all that natural sugar and fiber, I get a little water boost, so it's hydrating as well. Watermelon is great for that, too. Just about every morning I wake up and feel thirsty, so I eat a huge slice of ice-cold, crisp watermelon. It's so delicious! But then you know by now how much I love watermelon.

When I was running a lot every day, I would always want to eat something really wholesome because I saw it as an opportunity to get lots of great nutrients into my body. I'd have these big ole nut, berry, and dark lettuce salads that were so nutrient-rich that when I ate them I could feel them giving me power. I truly felt a strong sensation of my whole body absorbing that life-giving food. That's when you know your body is really working on the level it should be, instead of when you eat the kind of food that just sits there in the pit of your stomach, doing nothing much of anything.

As you know, one of my biggest temptations, sugar-wise, is pop. Coke is one of my favorite things in the whole world, and I can easily drink a couple of liters on ice. When we used to go out to eat, I would drink at least three Cokes—unless they only served Pepsi products, then I would enjoy a wheelbarrow full of icy Pepsi. It doesn't matter what the brand is, I just want that cold, dark, caffeinated sugar that makes my throat burn and my eyes water when I drink it. When I'm full and I'm eating my cheeseburger and fries, if I have a big sip of pop, it washes the food down and I can eat more. My thought process would be, *Well, my body is full, so I'm going to put this carbonated stuff into it to push the food down because we're still partying.*

It's gross when you think about it like that.

But drinking that much pop—or soda, depending on where you live—puts me way, way over the recommendations for how much added sugar I should be ingesting each day. To make that real, go to the kitchen and grab a teaspoon. Get the sugar out of the cupboard and find a glass. Now scoop out ten teaspoons of sugar into that glass. Quite a pile of white stuff there, right? That's how much sugar your average can of soda contains. Just to put that into perspective, the current recommendations are that as an adult man, I should consume nine teaspoons of sugar per day. Colette should have six teaspoons, and Gavin should have three teaspoons. With my three Cokes, I'm using up the daily allowance for a small family!

What does it matter? I hear you ask. An excellent question, my friend. It matters because not only does that extra sugar make us fat, there's also a strong and clear link between sugary drinks and diabetes. Say you're in the habit of drinking just one sugar-sweetened beverage, be it pop or a sweetened tea, each and every day. In ten years' time, your risk of developing diabetes will be 18 percent higher than your friend who regularly chooses ice water instead.

By now you're thinking that the solution is obvious. You should switch to diet sodas! Wrong, wrong, wrong. Studies also show a big connection between artificially sweetened drinks and a higher risk of diabetes. There is even a bunch of research that shows diet soda consumption over a period of time goes hand in hand with weight gain.

Just think: if everyone in the United States gave up drinking pop each day, by the year 2020, that single change would prevent two million new cases of diabetes. That's something to contemplate next time you reach for a fountain cup.

My thing now is that, when we go out to eat, I make a poor man's Sprite. I order a club soda, or Perrier, or Pellegrino—any bubbly water they have. If they don't have any, I just get them to spray soda water out of the tap and bring it to me. I'll squeeze two or three big limes straight into the glass and get as much lime juice in there as I can. Then I stir it up, and although it's not a Sprite, it still has the bubbles and the lime flavor, and it satisfies me. It's cold and it's refreshing.

Gavin did that last night, too, because he's been struggling with finding something to drink that feels fun, like pop.

SHAY: Did you find that it worked for you?

GAVIN: Yeah. When we used to go out to eat, I would get Sprite, but now I get seltzer with the limes. I like it with lots of ice so it's really cold, and I feel like it's more refreshing than a pop.

SHAY: I'm not going to tell you that kicking a soda habit is easy. Over the past week I've struggled really hard with the yearning to fill a cup with an icy-cold, bubbly, sweet beverage and knock it back. But giving up sugary drinks is at least achievable for everyone.

My local store has hardly any produce, people write to me. *If I want to buy fresh fruit and vegetables, I have to drive to the next town, ten miles away.* That can make it difficult, for sure. Not everyone has easy access to healthy foods. But here's a thing you can do that will save you money and improve your health. Sugar-sweetened drinks have zero health benefits, huge health risks, and they cost you money. There is no real down side to quitting soda; it's all upside—and I promise you'll never get a gold medal in deer-jumping if you're drinking buckets of caffeinated sugar twice a day.

Day 8

Be Like Spiderman

NOW THAT WE'VE been doing our challenge for over a week, I'm past the "detox" phase I described in an earlier chapter, and I'm starting to feel good.

I find that I don't need to sleep as much, and I think that's a side-effect of drinking plenty of water, eating healthy, and doing something active with Gavin every day. I even wake up when the sun comes up. Normally, I'd get up to use the bathroom and then go right back to bed—it's so easy to roll over and fall asleep again. But that doesn't work anymore, which kind of sucks. Now I find myself lying there for a while until I think, *Why don't I just get up?* It's annoying, in a way, but I'll get used to it. Having all this energy is a good thing.

I also feel thinner, although I haven't been weighing myself. I think people get too fixated on numbers—calories, minutes spent at the gym. In my experience, counting calories and hitting the gym is secondary to your attitude in determining your overall success. Sure, you might be able to follow a diet or rigorous exercise regimen in the short term, but if you have a negative attitude about it, if you dread it and resent everyone around you for living their lives, you won't be able to stick with it.

I think you're most vulnerable when you see someone having something you really, really want that you can't have. Yesterday afternoon, Emmi and Avia had piña-colada-flavored smoothies with whipped cream on top, and I could see Gavin watching them.

SHAY: Gavin, did you feel jealous? What were you thinking in that moment?

GAVIN: I didn't really feel jealous at all. I looked at it and thought, *I don't need that.* I reminded myself of our goals. And then I just forgot about it.

These are the kinds of moments that can throw you off from your goals. The thing is, you have the power to say, *Okay, this is happening. Getting mad or upset or jealous is a natural way to react, and I know most people would react that way. But I don't have to.* The decision is yours. You can say, *I'm not going to let it bother me.*

You know those movies or TV shows where they pause the action to show a character thinking through what they're going to do next? All the action stops while they work through their options. We do that every day, in a split second. Say someone walks into the room here and smacks me in the face. Between the time that dude hits me to the time I react, there's a moment in which I decide how to respond. The stimulus has no power over you in that moment, and that's why I call it the freedom zone.

It's not fair that my car broke down. It's not fair that guy smacked me in the face. It's not fair that my friends are all eating ice cream. Nothing is fair. We all have to deal with crap. But you choose how you react. Think of how much time you save by just moving on and being happy, rather than getting stuck in the "being mad" phase. That's what I admire about Gavin. When he saw his sisters drinking their piña colada smoothies, he chose to get over it. He didn't dwell on it. He told himself he didn't need one, and by thinking it, it became true. That considered choice, on top of other considered choices, will pay off in the long run.

You save time, you save stress, and all that crap that comes with being angry. All the stuff that could cause headaches, frustration, and sadness in your life suddenly doesn't mean a thing. It doesn't even exist, like Captain Atom has hit it with an energy blast.

This is the space in which people can choose to excel. The sooner you can make those choices, which are based on where you want to be in your life and the kind of person you want to be, the sooner you really claim that freedom zone. Every time a negative stimulus comes your way, pause and freeze time. You're like Spiderman with Doctor Octopus coming at you. Freeze the frame and think, *Stop. How am I going to react to this? I want to throw everything at him, but is that going to unleash more destruction?* Use that slice of time to make the best choice you can.

Oh, Shay, that's a cliché, people sometimes say to me. *You can't change your life just by deciding to change your life.* I feel so bad for people who think that, who really believe that they don't have 100 percent control over what they feel. Because I believe this wholeheartedly: you choose how you react to everything that happens to you. Of course you don't have control over what happens to you, and yes, people will do mean things to you. You will be treated unfairly. Trust me. It's life. Crappy things happen. But guess what? You choose how to react to that outside stimulus. Some of you believe that whatever those outside stimuli are, you are bound to feel a particular way in response. But you don't have to feel that way. You can say, *No. I'm in charge. I control what goes on here.*

The sooner you do that, I guarantee your life will get better.

Day 9

We Are Blood Brothers!

GAVIN AND I HAVE BEEN down in LA for a couple of days. I had to do some stuff for my digital production company, Maker Studios, and one of the things we decided for this challenge was that if I have to travel, Gavin has to come with me. We need to stick together on this—we're like blood brothers for these thirty days.

We did good in LA, and we ate well the whole time. We were near our favorite healthy food place, Rainbow Acres, so we drank a lot of juices. There were some temptations: we went out to dinner a lot, and we went to a Google-YouTube event; there was pop there, of course, and all kinds of stuff, but I don't think we messed up once.

Not eating sugar or highly processed foods cuts out 70 percent of everything in places like airports. It's all pop and candy and beef jerky and chips, so it gets hard to find anything to eat or drink. Same with gas stations—there are shelves and shelves of pop and candy and salty snack foods, and nothing healthy to be seen. Every time we go to a gas station, as soon as the kids see where we are, they all start calling out their orders. "I want gummy bears! I want a lemonade! I want this! I want that!" If we go to the gas station, we get treats for everybody. It's hard not to do that because it's fun. But that kind of thing can become commonplace, and a treat becomes what you do all the time. Is it still a treat then? I don't know.

Small changes make a difference. When I was thirteen or fourteen I did a similar challenge to Gavin's sugar diet that he did for a year. My mom told me that if I went for a year without candy and pop, she would give me a hundred bucks. It was just candy and pop—I could still eat other sugary things, like doughnuts. And it was a hundred bucks! I jumped on that, because we were poor and that was a lot of money to me.

Mom must have figured that it would be hard, but I did well for six months until my little brother Casey decided, *I'm going to get Shay*. So one day he poured Diet Coke into my orange juice to sabotage me. I remember drinking this glass of juice and screwing up my face, trying to figure out what the taste was. Casey got this big grin on his face and he started yelling, "Shay drank pop! Shay drank pop!"

Once I worked out what he had done, I started crying. "I didn't know! That's not fair!"

"It's all right, Shay," Mom told me. "Casey, stop it, you can't do that."

We still laugh about that story all the time. Mom forgave my half swig of Diet Coke–infused orange juice, and I ended up making it through the rest of the year and earning the one hundred bucks.

Yesterday we were talking about having access to fresh food, and it reminded me of when I was in fourth grade. Our family moved from Phoenix to Tremonton, a small town in Utah, for a year. They had the best school lunches in Tremonton. The lady who ran the cafeteria would bring in vegetables from her garden and serve up real homemade food every day. On one of my first days at school there, I took a bite out of something and said to the kid beside me, "What's with the food here?"

"What do you mean?" he asked me.

"Well . . . it's good!"

Even as a kid, it struck me what a difference it made, to come from a big school district to this smaller one. My new school had only two hundred kids or so, and the women in the cafeteria had the leeway to do what they wanted, so what they did was serve up this fantastic, nutrient-dense food.

Other than that year in Tremonton, I just remember school lunches being all about pizza and nachos and chocolate milk. Any vegetable options were frozen or from a can. Friday was peanut butter candy day at one school I went to. Then, when I was in high school, we had an open-campus policy for lunch, so we'd get in my friend Trevor Wight's truck and get lunch from some fast food-place. The exception was Wednesday, which was nachos day. My friend Jamey Jedrziewski and I would stay for lunch and eat this huge plate of nachos with cheese and sour cream, which was definitely not healthy.

Things have changed since then. In the past few years, there's been a huge amount of attention paid to what our kids eat at school. Around thirty million kids eat a school lunch every day, and that one meal can equal up to half their daily calories. So it matters what the schools dish up to them. Healthier foods can come as a shock when you're used to eating fast food and processed food. A bunch of kids tend to pick the items with the most sugar, like chocolate milk over plain, and they're used to the added flavor that sodium gives to food like canned vegetables. But there are simple ways to encourage better choices in the lunch line. Even setting out the healthy options first or putting plain milk in front of chocolate milk will make kids more likely to choose those things.

The changes still seem patchy, though, and there seems to be no rhyme or reason to whether kids get great lunches or super-processed food. When we lived in LA, the school Gavin attended a school in a very well-off area. You would think the parents would expect healthy options, but when I went up to the school, I was never that impressed with their food.

GAVIN: They would serve the food straight from the packages. I feel like the lunches we get in Idaho are better; maybe they're fresher. I still don't think they're really that healthy, though—usually we have two options, like a chicken burger or pizza, then you have to get at least one vegetable or fruit.

I would love to see every parent get behind a healthier lunch program. Nothing matters more than the future health of our children. I'm doing this healthy challenge with Gavin because I want him to learn better habits than I did growing up, and I know I'm not the only one who cares about seeing their children flourish into healthy, strong adults who know how to make good decisions for their lives.

Why stop at schools? Maybe they could make those same changes in public places, like ballparks and airports. I would love to see the concession stands at airports reinvented. Wherever there are racks of candy and pop and potato chips, replace them with racks of apples and bananas and snack-size bags of nuts. Tear down the burger concession and put in an organic salad bar. Install a juice bar where the booze bar is now. Forget the Bloody Mary, have a berry mango smoothie!

Maybe that can be the next thing Gavin and I do together, after writing this book. Oh yeah, I can see it now: Shay and Gavin's Fly Fresh Airport Concessions. Watch this space . . .

Day 10

Fattest Weight-Loss Expert Ever

I don't like to run. But let's say I had a soccer ball that I had to dribble. I could probably go, like, eight miles! You're so distracted by trying to dribble the ball, so you aren't thinking about how far you've gone or how much more you have to go. Your mind focuses on the ball.

We're still in LA, so yesterday Gavin and I went down to the beach and played some beach soccer. Running on sand is the best workout ever. I can't recommend it enough. It makes your legs and feet so strong—it's like running with weights strapped to your ankles! You really have to use your whole body, from your toes to your shoulders. Beach soccer is so intense, like interval training. You have to do a lot of short bursts of activity, which works your body in a different way than a long-drawn-out run. Man, you know you've had a real workout after running around on the sand for thirty minutes.

We were going to explore the rocks, but we got yelled at by the lifeguard. He whistled at us and told us to get out of the water, but as we started to walk out, he kept whistling and pointing. We were like, *Dude, we know, we're getting out. Leave us alone. We're two buff dudes running on the beach, we can handle ourselves.*

I acknowledge that there's a faint possibility that the lifeguard *might* not have seen us as two buff dudes.

Here's a tweet I got when I started my father-son challenge with Gavin:

> *Shay, you're the fattest weight-loss expert I've ever seen.*

Another one simply said:

> *Here we go again.*

It's true that I'm not that guy on the cover of *Muscle & Fitness* magazine, with my rippling six-pack and my gleaming biceps. I am not that guy, I admit it. What I am is the guy who tries, and succeeds, then finds himself sliding back into old, unhealthy habits, so he needs to find new ways to try again. And again. And again.

Yes, you're right: here we go again. But I'm not going to stop doing that, no matter what anyone says to me.

I've never claimed to be an expert; I'm just a regular dude trying to lose weight and get in shape, and trying to bring his son along on the journey to find healthier ways to live his life. Regular dudes fail. They mess up and have to start over again.

When it comes to weight loss, I'm probably as well known for my failures as my successes. Back in 2009, I lost over a hundred pounds by working hard, following a raw food diet, and training to run my first-ever marathon—and then going on to run two more. At that point in my life, I felt on top of the world; I was unstoppable. But after about three years, the weight crept back on: I stopped exercising so intensely, I indulged myself in fast food and desserts and sodas, and before I knew it I had gained back about twenty of those pounds. So if I'm an expert at anything, it's about dealing with failure.

When I say "failure," it's not like I've totally crashed since that first big weight-loss effort. I didn't regain all of that hundred-plus pounds, just a relatively small chunk of it. I'm still exercising; I just lost some of the fire along the way.

I have things that I need to work on: I'm more acutely aware of that than anyone else in the room. It's important to me to be open about the times I mess up as well as the times I get it right, and I have always documented those moments on YouTube. There are videos where I have opened up and said, "I know there are things that I need to do that I haven't been doing, or I haven't pushed as hard as I need to because I'm lazy. Now I want to make a recommitted effort to do those things."

All too often, the reaction I get is, *It's not going to happen. You're not going to do it, Shay. You're all talk.* When people say those things, I wonder what they're saying about themselves inside their own minds, and if they're projecting some of their own issues onto me. Because, let's face it, we all struggle with fear of failure. The ShayLoss journey is all about working together as a team and feeling good because we're working together—just like Gavin and I are working together through this month. And yet the first thing some people want to do is tear others down.

If that's you, I've got to wonder—who else in your life is doing that to you? Maybe your parents say things that are discouraging.

Mom, Dad, I'm going to do this.

No, you're not. You're not going to do that. You can't do that.

Maybe because you experience that in your life, you bring it over to YouTube. You've got to be able to change that mind-set. You've got to be able to be honest with yourself, sit down, and say, "Is that the reason why I'm like this? I don't like that. I want to change it." That's the first step: allowing yourself to admit the things that you need to work on.

Some of you won't be able to admit those things. There might even be things that I need to admit to. What are they? One is that I get really excited about a new project or an idea, and then burn myself out. After I ran the St. George Marathon, I didn't feel the fire like I did after my first marathon. You know why? It's because I got burned out. I pushed that thing so hard. I ran twenty-six miles in three hours and eleven minutes. That's pretty dang fast. It's great, and I'm proud of that achievement, but if I'm honest with myself, every time I have thought about doing another marathon since that race, it just seems too painful to contemplate.

Something needs to be different, though, and this time the difference is doing a challenge with—and for—my son Gavin. This is not the same old routine, because this time I'm driven to make a change for his sake. On top of that, I'm straight-up tired of carrying around extra weight. When I'm making the end slates of the Shaytards vlogs, I look back at myself a year or two ago, and I remember how good I felt then. How did I ever let myself slip back into this chubby, sedentary lifestyle? "Sedentary" might be overstating it, because I have been lifting weights, but I can't go out and run fifteen miles right now, and I miss that. I'm sick and tired of being sick and tired, so I'm making a change.

Sure, the changes I make are extreme. *You're yo-yo dieting*, people say. To me I just go hard—and then I stop going so hard. Moderation is something that doesn't come easy to me, so I try to find ways to live a better life that work for me and who I am.

We all have our flaws and our failings. Weight loss doesn't exist in its own little box, separate from the rest of your life. It's all part and parcel of the same picture: the attitudes you bring to your marriage, to your job, to your kids, to your parents, to your friends will all turn up in your weight-loss journey.

That's why I say this is not a diet book. This is not just about what you put in your mouth, or whether you lace up your running shoes today. This is about your life, every joyful, messy, painful, delightful part of it. And we're in it together, dudes.

Day 11

———

Five Cinnamon Rolls Please

CAN YOU BELIEVE we're eleven days in—more than a third of the way through our challenge?! I feel like I'm getting used to doing without the sugar, and making sure we get some exercise every day. Meeting our water goal is still hard a lot of the time—I just forget to drink enough. But I'm feeling good.

Gavin is definitely looking better. We got a lot of great exercise in LA by playing soccer on the beach, and then we came back to the mountains of Idaho and went on a trek, pushing handcarts in the hot sun for seven and a half miles. We were definitely hurting the next day! We also just got one of those big aboveground pools, so Gavin has been slipping and sliding and jumping into the pool with his cousins—we had eight hundred and one cousins over here the other night for Brock's birthday. So it's definitely summertime go-time.

SHAY: Gavin, do you feel better? Have you noticed a difference?

GAVIN: Yeah. I notice that I used to not run very fast, but yesterday I beat Cooper. I couldn't believe that our challenge was actually working.

Cooper is Gavin's cousin. He's younger than Gavin, but this kid is seriously athletic. So for Gavin to beat him in a footrace is great.

You know, it feels good to be doing something. Anything would be better than living the kind of unhealthy lifestyle we were living before. Last night, I was looking back at the video we shot for my amazingly beautiful wife Colette's thirty-second birthday, when the whole Butler family went to Disneyland to celebrate, and it reminded me of how this book came about.

"Five large Mickey Mouse cinnamon rolls please." As soon as those words were out of my mouth a voice inside my head shouted, *You have to write a weight-loss book, Shay!* You know those voices, right? They're the same ones that say to you:

How many hours can you really spend on Netflix?

When are you going to do your homework?

You shouldn't stay up so late!

You should wake up early!

You know, the voices that always want to ruin all the fun.

But like I always do in these "you're doing something that you probably shouldn't be doing" situations, I had multiple justifications ready to present to those shouting voices inside my head that would question the wisdom of ordering five towering mountains of frosting that average around 2,500 calories apiece. Colette had just given birth to Daxton—our fifth perfectly healthy child—seven months earlier, and currently looked like she could pass for a twenty-two-year-old. If having a beautiful family and a gorgeous wife celebrating her birthday wasn't reason enough to be splurging at Mickey's magical wonderland, then take this into consideration: I'm a cofounder of Maker Studios, *a company that had just been sold to the Walt Disney Corporation for close to $1 billion.*

A company that I had helped launch five years earlier in Venice Beach, California, had been sold to one of the—if not *the*—biggest entertainment and media companies to ever exist on the face of the globe, just mere days before Colette's birthday. The story was on the front page of my hometown paper the *Idaho State Journal.* That's a big deal where I come from. It was also in thousands of other newspapers: the *New York Times,* the *Wall Street Journal, USA Today,* the *Los Angeles Times, Variety, The Guardian* in the UK, *Billboard, Hollywood Reporter.* It was on the lips of everybody in my industry. I had won the proverbial "Disney Lottery." Indeed, it was a dream come true—a dream I never knew I even had! And finally, we were standing in the very location that millions upon millions of people from around the world commonly refer to as "the happiest place on Earth."

We had been to Disneyland many times over the last five years, and we even had season passes two of those five years. In fact, some of our best and most-viewed videos were ones showing our whole family on the rides there. But this time it was different. This was the first time that I had been to the park since the purchase of the company I had cofounded. This place that encourages dreaming had literally granted me the greatest wish I never knew was imaginable. Disneyland had made me a millionaire!

If anybody had the right to order five plates of warm, creamy, steaming cellulite from the organization that taught him that dreams really do come true, it was me.

Whenever the Shaytards go anywhere, it's usually in a pack of children. For starters, Colette and I have five kids, and we often hang out with my siblings or Colette's, who also have multiple children. When we're all out in a public place together, we look like a day care on a field trip. I've seen the look of terror on far too many hostesses' faces when I utter the words "We need ten kids' menus please." So on this particular day, we wrestled our plethora of hungry, excited children to the dining area as I proudly carried in both hands two red plastic trays that were buckling under the weight of my five delicious heaps of diabetes. I couldn't wait to take my first bite!

As I gently placed as much cinnamon roll creaminess as one thirty-four-year-old man with average dexterity can fit onto one standard-size amusement park plastic fork, I delivered one final piece of rationalization to those voices inside my head. This last great justification would drive my point home and act as a nail in the coffin for those voices seeking to question my deathly delicious five-cinnamon-roll decision. It's a line that all great procrastinators use. Maybe you've heard it? Maybe you've used it yourself? It's almost considered cliché because of how much it's used, but I was for real this time: "The diet starts tomorrow!"

Yes, that phrase that saves us all from doing the dreaded hard thing now. The phrase that lets us indulge in that one last deliciousness, because tomorrow is the day that we're going to get serious about having a healthy body. And I was really serious this time. Summer was coming and I had just signed a deal to write my very first book. It was supposed to be about weight loss, but here I was, ordering enough calories to add a third and even a fourth chin to my chubby neckline. But I didn't want to think about that right now. Today was a celebration. We were at *Disneyland*!

This was also meant to be a last hoorah to a job well done. We were moving back home to Idaho the very next day. I felt overwhelming gratitude and was overjoyed at what it meant for our family to move back to the land of potatoes. This was our last sunny, Southern California sunset, and I wanted to *par-tay*!

But the truth is, as I sat on that beautifully lit, well-cleaned veranda, serenaded by Mary Poppins singing those immortal words "Just a spoonful of sugar helps the medicine go down, in a most delightful way," surrounded by my loved ones all battling for the middle of that molten mountain of greasy goo, and as I took that first bite, I couldn't help but admit that I felt like crap. Not because I wasn't deliriously happy and thankful for a Mount Everest's worth of blessings, but my body felt like crap, and when your body feels like crap, *you* feel like crap!

I had gained a good chunk of blue whale blubber in the last six months. I was at that point where my favorite pair of jeans, which were once upon a time the coolest and most comfortable pair of pants I owned, were now more of a "tummy tourniquet." Have you ever worn pants that are so tight your legs go numb? So tight you get a stomachache after wearing them, but you suffer through it because *gosh dangit* I'm a thirty-four-inch waist, and I am *not* shopping for forty-eight inchers in the "big and bigger" section of the local Walmart ever again!

As I slowly shoveled another tasty morsel of chewy chunkiness into the two-inch hole in my face, I felt a hand on my shoulder and heard the voice of my younger brother Casey say, "What you thinking about, big guy?"

"Do people who order five cinnamon rolls write good weight-loss books?" I asked him.

He cackled his high-pitched laugh that makes me smile every time I hear it. My brother Casey is hilarious to me. He can make me laugh harder than anyone I know. Just one year and seven months apart, we grew up as best friends and fellow daredevils. We were the crazy kids in our neighborhood. We jumped off cliffs, skated on ramps, built zip lines in our trees, skipped school, and skied every chance we could. We also, allegedly, threw dirt clods at oncoming cars driving down the brand-new road that was constructed directly over the open field where we built our BMX bike jumps. (Only allegedly, Mom—but it was Casey's fault!) We were always up to something. I bet we burned three thousand calories a day. We were having fun, not "working out." Our bodies were finely tuned machines, designed for riding moguls on our skis, doing backflips off diving boards, and sprinting from the scene of a freshly toilet-papered house. I missed that feeling!

As I wiped a smear of icing off my beard, I decided then and there: it was time to make a change.

Inside my head I uttered those immortal words: "The diet starts—tomorrow."

Day 12

Let's Flippin' Do This!

YOU THINK GOLF isn't great exercise? That it's just a gentle little amble across the grass? Not the way we played it this past weekend. Gavin and I went golfing, and he kept doing these dinky little shots that went fifteen yards. Every time he did that, I would tell him to go get it, so he would sprint over and grab the ball then run back. He was running a ton, so playing golf that way is definitely good exercise.

After we finished, we had a big father-son talk about this book. Gavin and I both know that at the end of the day, we have to show results. People are going to expect us to have lost weight. But I don't want to harp on about it, and I sure don't want Gavin to hate that we have to do this—to hate me because he thinks, *Dad's nagging on me about losing weight.*

We all have to be accountable to ourselves and be committed to our lives and our bodies and how we feel. Each of us has to find that power inside, whether we're kids or grown-ups.

After that conversation, Gavin was kind of quiet. The next morning, I asked him what he was thinking about it all, and he read out to me what he had written in his journal.

I'm excited about the book. Thanks to you, Dad, I can and I will do anything and put my mind to it. Thanks, Dad. Let's flippin' do this.

That seriously made me choke up a little bit, because that's how I feel, too. I'm excited and I want to do this—not just for myself, but for my family, which matters to me more than anything in this world. It's my love for my kids that actually brought me to YouTube in the first place.

When I first got married, I was over the moon excited. I was in the deepest love I could imagine with my little brunette named Colette. I had known I wanted to marry her from the very first day I saw her. So now that we were eternally sealed together in holy matrimony, I *knew* she was mine! This may sound a little bit crazy, but for months after our wedding, I would think to myself, *Holy crap, I can't believe she actually married me.* It was like knowing that you would have your dream girlfriend forever and she could never break up with you . . .

Okay, this is starting to sound creepy.

Anyway, one morning, after we had been married for a few weeks, I saw Colette taking some pills. "What's that you're taking?" I asked her.

"My birth control," she replied.

It surprised me when she said it because I hadn't really given much thought to babies or starting a family. Those were things that were always far away in the future. I had been focused on persuading this girl to marry me. I always wanted to be a father and always assumed I would have three or four kids, but in typical dude fashion I never really gave it much thought. Colette and I had talked a few times about having kids, but now that I was actually married, that conversation was getting a lot more serious.

We sat there and talked about it, right then and there. But this conversation wasn't like all of the others. It was more along the lines of, "Do you want to have kids . . . right now?" A "What if we threw away the birth control and made a baby right now?" kind of conversation. Those are serious conversations! I had absolute zero insight into what having a baby would entail, but I thought that it sounded fun. So I said, "Let's have a baby!"

Nine months later, Gavin Shay Butler was born. I was a dad!

The only problem with being a dad when you've never been a dad before is that you don't know how to be a dad. I knew that I wanted to be a good dad, though, and I would do whatever it took to figure it out.

When you first become a dad, the main thing on your mind is providing for your wife and child. I knew if there was one thing that I was definitely in charge of as husband and father of this little family, it was to earn money for food and shelter.

By the time Gavin was born, we had lived barely ten months as adults in the real world. The honeymoon was over. We had rent and bills and student loans. I had already experienced what it felt like to be at a supermarket and watch your wife take things off the conveyor belt and put them back because the total on the register was larger than the amount in our checkbook. Now that we had a baby, I couldn't imagine the horror of Colette not being able to buy diapers or food because we didn't have money. So that became my main focus. How do I make more money? How do I provide for my family?

Like most husbands and fathers, I went to work. I went to a *lot* of work. It wasn't unusual for me to spend fifty, sixty hours a week working. That means I was only seeing my brand-new baby maybe a couple of hours a day. Little Gavin was usually asleep when I left in the mornings and in bed or going to bed when I got home in the evenings. So during the week, I was hardly ever spending time with the person that I was doing all the work for in the first place!

I often say that the reason I quit college was because I couldn't find a parking spot. Every time I went to this one particular class, my psychology class, there were never any parking spots. Avia, our second child, had just been born, so my wife and my two children were at home, and I'd be circling around, trying to find somewhere to park after having spent $140 on a book my professor wrote, and after I found somewhere to park, I'd just be sitting there, listening to this guy's opinion, having just spent a whole lot of money to buy a book with the same thing in it. Then next year he'd write a revised edition, so I'd be able to sell the book he just sold to me, except I'd get fifteen bucks for it, and I'd have to buy his new book for $160. All so I could get three points toward a certificate that says I can have a job. BULL CRAP!

Screw that, I decided. *I'm going to start working on my own. I don't need these guys to tell me when I can start living in the real world.* So I dropped out of college and never looked back. That was the right decision for me. But kids, go to college. If you don't know what you're going to do, you should go there until you figure it out.

It's not like I'd never worked before in my life. That's the one thing my dad taught me growing up. I would always remember him saying, "You need to learn how to work." He taught me how to work, and I worked a lot of different jobs. Dishwashing was probably the worst. When I was sixteen, I was a dishwasher at this steak and seafood restaurant. The older cooks liked to mess with the new guys, so they would slam me at eleven o'clock at night. They'd bring me all their broiler trays, grease traps, and oven hood vents, and I'd be there scrubbing these things until two in the morning.

I wasn't afraid of working hard, but I wanted to do something with purpose, so I never settled into any of the jobs I had. All that time, I was searching for a career. I had a great wife and wonderful kids. But I wanted to know, what am I going to do with my life? What's my career going to be? We moved all over the place while I worked different jobs. I've been a car salesman. I've been a real estate agent. I've sold pest control door to door. We lived in North Carolina, Phoenix, and Dallas. At one point I started my own granite business called Rock Tops, and I'd drive around town with a truck with magnets on it that I'd designed myself. I felt proud that I had started my own business, but I didn't like it and I knew I wouldn't do it forever.

When I was at the granite shop, though, the seeds of a life in entertainment were planted. Hard to imagine how that could happen, right? Stay with me on this one. On Z103, the radio station we used to listen to in the granite shop, they had a trivia segment called "The Answer's Never Dirty." The morning disc jockeys would ask a question that sounded like the answer could be dirty, but it wasn't. Something like, "Thirty percent of women like this in bed," and the answer would be silk sheets. For some reason, we called in one day, and the first answer was a total guess. I couldn't even remember what the question was, so we said "croquet," as in the game of croquet, as our answer. Then we kept calling and saying the answer was "croquet" every day.

"Who is this?" the radio DJ would say.

"Oh, it's Shay calling."

"Hey, it's Croquet Shay!"

The question might've been, "How many people do this in their spare time?" And I'd say, "Read *Croquet Weekly.*"

Finally, the radio DJ said, "If you stop calling in and doing this, I'll give you your own segment on Wednesdays."

This segment was called "Doghouse Wednesday." People would call in when they were in trouble with their wife or husband. Three people would tell their stories, then I would judge who was in the biggest doghouse. It was fun. I would yell at them: "What were you thinking?!" and one of them would win a trip somewhere.

I got to know the program director at the radio station pretty well, so when they were hiring a weekend DJ, I called him up.

"Hey, Brad, I want to do that. I want to be the DJ on the weekends."

"Okay," he said, "you've been on the radio for six months now anyway." That was technically true, though I had never gone in to the station—I just called in on the phone. So he gave me the job and I did weekends. Then I got my own show; I was on Monday through Friday from six to midnight. I loved that job. It was fun thinking on my feet, hearing cool music, and taking phone calls. I started doing live shows on Blog TV from the radio station as I was broadcasting. It was like working with two separate audiences at the same time: I was talking to people who were watching me live on the Internet at the same time as I was deejaying for an entirely different audience.

It never dawned on me that I could grow up and become an entertainer. That never seemed realistic. I never thought, *Oh, I'll grow up to be an entertainer!* What did that even mean? I can't really sing, I'm not an actor, and I'm not a stand-up comedian. The very first time the idea was put into my head was by a very good friend of mine named Jamey—the same guy I'd eaten nachos with on Wednesdays in high school. At his wedding, I got to give a toast in front of two hundred people, and I had the whole crowd cracking up. Afterward, when I was leaving, I said to Jamie, "Hey, congratulations!" and as I was hugging him, he said to me, "Dude, you've got to get your comedy out there!"

What do you mean, "get my comedy out there"? I was thinking. *What comedy to get out where? How would I even go about that?*

My radio work gave me a glimmer of an idea of how that could happen, but the pieces really came together when I was twenty-seven. Our third child, Emmi, had just been born, and I was working in the granite shop, doing my radio gig on the side. Colette and I had just bought a house, and one day I said to her, "Honey, should we get a computer?"

"What will we use it for?" she asked me.

"I don't know, maybe to send emails or something."

I had never owned a computer. I did start a typing class, but because I hadn't taken the prerequisite class, they kicked me out. And frankly, I was terrible. The only two things I'd ever done on a computer were have a Hotmail account and play Oregon Trail.

The next day, I went out and bought myself a little Dell laptop for five hundred bucks. I got home and opened it up. *Whoa, this thing is awesome.*

Late at night, around eleven p.m., I started playing on it. Colette had gone to bed, and I was sitting on this little desk chair we have in our bedroom. "All right, honey, I'll be in bed in a second." I was just looking around, and somehow I stumbled on to YouTube.

Because I used to ski a lot, I love ski tricks, so I was watching all these ski videos. Then I thought, *Oh, I love Green Day*, so I checked out a Green Day concert. I just started typing in all these things I wanted to see, and I was sitting in this little hard chair watching YouTube videos, and I looked out the window and saw that the sun had risen. I had stayed up all night long watching YouTube videos. I stood up, freaking out. *Are you kidding me?*

From that first night of watching YouTube videos all night long, I was hooked. Then I put up a few videos of my own: little videos I had made just for fun but hadn't planned to put on YouTube. I had a few videos of me dancing in a unitard, and one of me skiing, and a video during my mom's fiftieth birthday party of my brothers and me sucking helium from a balloon. They got zero views.

Then I noticed that people on YouTube had schedules and shows. The first person I subscribed to was Dax Flame, who's kind of controversial. If you haven't seen him, he's truly funny: he made a series of vlogs showing himself as a socially awkward fifteen-year-old, and no-one was sure if it was clever acting or the real deal. There were thousands of comments debating this point on each of his videos.

Wow, there are thousands of people sitting here talking about this guy, I thought. *It would be fun to do something like that.*

Next, I started watching Phil DeFranco, who went by the YouTube name sxephil, and I noticed that he had a regular show three days a week. *This dude has an Internet show, and he's just a regular guy. I could do that.* He held a contest, and I entered it with a concept about a he-man germ. There's this antibacterial soap that says it kills 99.9 percent of germs. My line was, "What about that .01 percent? That's the he-man germ. He's the germ I want dead." I did this whole rant on that, and Phil DeFranco picked it as one of the finalists, so I got a shout-out from Phil on his channel.

Things snowballed: I started getting subscribers, some dude from Nebraska emailed me saying I should make more videos, I got more emails, and I got more subscribers. It seemed so weird and crazy, but the connection was almost addictive. Before I went to bed at night, I'd upload a video. Then when I woke up in the morning, I was so excited to read the comments and see what people were saying.

Everything really took off when I started daily vlogs. When I turned twenty-nine, I said to myself, *This is the last year of my twenties. I want to do something cool for this year—because I'm not going to be twenty-something anymore, I'm going to be friggin' thirty!*

It was a quarter-life crisis, I guess you could say. So I decided to make a YouTube video every single day for the last year of my twenties. At the time, nobody was doing that—all my other YouTube friends were making two or three a week.

"Well, you think I should try to upload a video every day?" I asked them.

"I don't know, that sounds crazy," people said.

That settled it. "I'm going to do it."

So on March 5, 2009, I started uploading a video every single day. Because you get paid to upload videos, the more videos you upload, the more you get paid. After a month of daily videos, I could see the pay definitely getting better. *We could live off this and I won't have to do granite anymore*, I figured.

The very last granite job I ever did was for my little brother, Casey. He bought a house, and I did his granite in his kitchen. I said, "Okay, this is the last manual labor job I'm ever doing. I'm done with it. I'm going to work smarter, not harder." And that's how it all began.

So when I say I started out doing YouTube for my family, I also mean that wider family, the community of people that I'm connected with. And when I talk about doing YouTube, I'm talking about the whole of it: the ShayLoss videos, the challenges, the workouts. Which brings me back to why Gavin and I are writing this book—for the same reason: for that great big family we're all in together.

Day 13

The Magical Secret Life Ingredient

IT'S TIME FOR a reset. We're thirteen days in now, and the water is not working. Gavin hates drinking the gallon of water. The first couple of days, I would give him the gallon, and he would drink half of it. "Dude," I'd say, "you have to finish your water." And he'd say, "It tastes gross."

SHAY: Yeah, but I finished it.
GAVIN: That's true. But we can find some ways to make it easier.

There have been some days we haven't drunk a full gallon, so we decided to really push it for seven days in a row. We went down to the grocery store and bought fourteen gallons of water and lined them up on a shelf in our garage. We have a fridge down there, too, so we have a four-gallon rotation to keep the ones we're drinking cold.

It's hard to drink water when it gets warm. Gavin likes his drinks seriously cold—he even chews on ice. He'll fill a big glass of crushed ice and pour in the water, then he'll chew the ice after he's done drinking. Problem is, we don't have a crushed icemaker. We just bought a big, fancy new fridge and it doesn't crush the ice. What a piece of crap.

If we duct tape our gallon water jugs to our hands and we can't untape them until we're done drinking—maybe that'll work? Hmm.

When I wake up in the morning, I often feel thirsty, but I'm looking around for a cup or a bottle; if it's not right there, I simply don't end up drinking water. It needs to be there in the same way we have snacks on hand for that mindless snacking that most of us do. Because we've got so many kids around the place, we always have something in the house to snack on—chips and salsa, cookies, or Pop-Tarts. I want to replace that with something better, and if I have my gallon jug with me all the time, whether I'm riding my bike or editing some videos, I'll be halfway done drinking it before I know it, just because it's there. Mindless drinking, if you will.

Water is a magical secret life ingredient, so it yields huge dividends if you drink loads of it. I always, always, always feel so much better waking up on a morning when I drink a ton of water the night before. Drinking a ton of water before bed, even if you have to pee in the middle of the night and it's a little inconvenient, allows you to wake up feeling so much better.

Your body needs more water than you believe it does. Our bodies are 55 to 60 percent water. Can you imagine that? That's what the doctors and the scientists say, but I have a hard time believing it—wouldn't that make us like giant jellyfish walking around, driving our cars, mowing the lawn? But if our bodies really are made up of a majority of water, it makes sense that we need to maintain them by consuming a lot of water. That's why fruits and vegetables are so good for you: they're also mainly water, so you're putting into your body exactly what it craves.

You've got to pace yourself, though. Watch that clock. You don't want to be chugging down the last half of a gallon of water right before bedtime, because you'll have to wear a diaper. Try and drink a good amount early in the day. Your body works in cycles: your sleep cycles between REM and non-REM sleep, and your body is attuned to the cycle of daylight, to awake when the sun rises. You're supposed to eat during the day and then digest at night, then the next morning, from when you wake up until noon, is the elimination cycle. I don't want to gross you out, but that's when you poop and pee and get all of the waste products out of your body.

Early in the day is when exercise and water are the most valuable, because your body is trying to get rid of all the previous day's waste. As you exercise in the morning, you burn all of the stuff that is left over, and then as you drink water, your body is able to use it to flush the waste out of your system. By lunchtime, you should feel pretty good because you're all flushed out, you're hydrated, and you're ready to eat a high-nutrient lunch. You eat that lunch and you feel *good*.

That's how it should go, anyway. But the norm for many of us is that you get up, you're tired, you buy your Starbucks loaded with sugar and caffeine, then you eat a McMuffin or something. Your body is still trying to get rid of all of the stuff from the day before, then all of a sudden you're putting this sugar and bread inside of yourself. For your body, it feels like this: *Man, I've still got all of this stuff from last night—now I have to process all of this new stuff. Okay, I'm going to have to focus completely on dealing with this right now.*

By noon, you're feeling like you just want to go back to bed. Your body is maxed out.

That's why it's so important to help your body eliminate all of that stuff in the morning so that by lunchtime it can say, *I'm ready to eat again, give me some good healthy fuel.* When you give it the water and the nutrients it's calling out for, your body gives you the power to propel you through a day of work, right through to five o'clock when you can go home to your family. Drinking water the whole day just keeps you going.

Today Dad and I talked about how our bodies are like conveyor belts. Every day boxes come on the conveyor belt and you have to break them down so they're flat, then after you break down a box you stack it on a pile on the side. But one day you're breaking down boxes and all of a sudden a bunch of boxes are coming in and you're racing and racing to get the boxes broken down. Pretty soon you start throwing unbroken-down boxes to the side and you start storing

them. Sometimes-or hopefully most
of the time-paper boxes come in and
they're easy to break down. Those
represent fruits and vegetables. But
sometimes plastic boxes come on the
conveyor belt and they're hard to break
down-they represent junk food. So we
want to put the paper boxes in our body.

The way I figure it, our bodies are like a factory production line. Boxes are sent down the line and workers are busy breaking them down and folding them flat. On a good day, our bodies work away, folding the boxes, keeping on top of it all. But on a bad day, too many boxes come down the conveyor belt, and maybe some of them are made out of plastic so they're hard to break down. The system gets overloaded. There's panic, things start to back up, and some boxes are set over to the side to deal with later.

So when I grab that extra handful of flesh around my stomach, that's my box storage area. When we send food down our throats and into our intestines, it may be the kind of food that's easy to break down because it's of a similar constitution to our bodies, being 60 percent water. Or it may be highly processed food that takes longer to break down into its components. When there's a lot of that kind of food coming down the line, or simply too much food in total, that's when your storage area expands.

The math is simple: You just have to break down all of the boxes that are coming down the conveyor belt. If you're sending down the wrong kind of boxes or too many of them, you're going to have that extra fat around your waist.

One thing that always frustrates me with weight loss is that I want results like *that* (I'm snapping my fingers here, can you hear that?). This is probably true for anybody: you go three or four days and it seems so tough and you think, *I'm dying here, and I've only lost one pound.* It's so tempting to keep checking those scales, but I'm here to say, don't weigh yourself a lot because it can have the opposite effect from the encouragement you need right now. Change is going to happen over a long period of time.

What keeps me going mentally is seeing results. I don't believe in jumping on the scales every ten seconds, but I do like to weigh myself once a week. I weighed in this morning and found out that a couple of pounds of me have been sucked into the universe! I'm feeling great and it's motivating to know that I'm doing it this time. Lots of times I've said I would get healthy again and I didn't do it, but I feel like I'm really committed this time; I can feel the commitment there in my mind. It's making a huge difference to be doing this challenge with Gavin. I know I can't let him down because we're in this together.

One of my favorite quotes is from the movie *Shawshank Redemption.* Andy Dufresne is a banker who is accused of murder and does time in Shawshank prison. While he's there, he makes friends with an older guy called Red. After Andy tunnels his way out of Shawshank, Red says that he would have thought it was impossible, but Andy loves geology, which is the study of time and pressure. That's all it takes, Red says: pressure and time. Andy had the time and he kept applying the pressure, and he dug that giant tunnel out of the prison. It's the same with weight loss. It's all about continued time and pressure. You can't make big changes just like *that* (I'm snapping my fingers again here). You've got to keep focusing and keep pushing day by day by day. All of a sudden, two weeks have gone by, and you've lost ten pounds. All of a sudden a month's gone by, and you've lost twenty pounds. You've got to keep going, keep going, keep going.

Don't get frustrated with the time. Just keep pushing on.

And don't accuse me of promoting bad influences, like guys who broke out of prison. Andy was innocent!

Day 14

I Adopted a Million Children!

GAVIN IS REALLY starting to see the difference in how his body behaves. Yesterday we played football with his sisters and their cousins, seven kids in total. I was all-time quarterback because I've got a great arm; I could throw a football over a mountain if I needed to. We made this rule that if you caught the ball, you got to go again, and if you stopped a player, then they could be the receiver. That motivated the kids to play good defense, because all the kids wanted to be the person to catch the ball. Gavin was hustling hard. He was getting open, outrunning Avia and his cousin Brailey. There were two occasions where Gavin caught the ball five times in a row, and the other kids were complaining that they weren't getting to be the receiver because

Gavin kept catching it. We had to make a five-catch cap: you could only catch it five times in a row and then you had to be on defense and somebody else got a turn.

I could tell he was winded, but he wanted to keep going because he was competing with his cousins. Two of his cousins are a couple of years younger than him, but they're pretty athletic, and Brailey is just a little younger than him. It was all of them against Gavin, so he was really hustling. It was clear that he has become quicker and more agile. I don't think he could have out-juked all those kids before.

Seeing him in action, knowing that his body is able to do more things now, is an incomparable feeling. Way beyond the numbers on the scale, this is what it's all about.

Doing a challenge by yourself is hard, no doubt about it. Before we started this one, I figured that it would be good for Gavin and me to do it together; it would make us healthier, bring us closer together as father and son. What I didn't predict was that he would be such a great motivator.

I feel like he has been good competition. He's definitely doing better than I am at some things. With the water, for example, I'll say to him, "Let me see your jug," and he'll have drunk more than me. *Dang, I need to catch up*, I'll think.

Your family has such power to lift you up or bring you down. I'm the person I am largely because of my wife. Colette has been so supportive throughout the years—not only with getting into YouTube, but before that, when I was still casting around to find what I should do with my life. When I wanted to move to North Carolina to be a door-to-door pest control salesman, she supported me. We lived in Idaho at the time, and she could so easily have said, *What? We're going to move to the East Coast to sell pest control? That's crazy, no way we're going to do that!* But she always believed in me, and we've always made it work. There were times when we had to have those conversations that went, "Do we pay the gas bill or do we save this money for groceries because we don't have any food in the house?" As a newly-wed couple and then later as parents with young children, those times were definitely hard.

Making money out of YouTube wasn't instantaneous, by any means. I was uploading videos for a little while before I started making any money at all, but once I finally got partnered I could see that I was making money. Once you're linked, you have an AdSense account where you can see how much you're making. One morning, I logged on and there were two or three dollars in the account. I couldn't believe it. *Whoa, when I upload this video, this thing with the money goes up a little bit. Holy crap!* Making that connection was so cool. For a month's worth of videos, we got $326. We could pay our light bill and our water bill with that!

At first, it was all about getting a little extra money in to help pay our bills. We had just bought a house and our mortgage payment was one thousand bucks a month, so I set myself a goal: to make one thousand bucks a month out of YouTube so that we could make that mortgage payment. Well, we reached that goal. Then one day I realized that I was making enough out of YouTube to replace my regular income, and that this was my new job. That was when I quit everything else and just started doing YouTube.

YouTube has been a perfect medium for me to fall into. That idea of "getting my comedy out there" and being an entertainer came about through that evolution. This makes sense: this is me. People who have known me all my life will tell you, *Oh, that's just Shay being Shay.* Once I made the switch to entertaining people, first on radio and then on YouTube, I never looked back. I want this to be my career, and it's worked so far. Out of all the jobs I've had, being a full-time YouTuber is the longest job I've ever had. This is what I do.

Even now, it's the freedom that matters most: being able to spend time with my wife and my kids. If you were to say, *I will give you a billion dollars but you have to work nine to five, Monday through Friday, at this place, and you have to do exactly what I tell you to do*, I'd say, *No way.* I'm not going to do it because freedom is more valuable to me than the money. Colette and I are able to make enough money to provide for our family. Even if I could make substantially more money some other way, losing that freedom is not worth it.

More than the money, I feel like I've adopted about a million children now. All of the people who have subscribed feel like family. There are some people who have been on this journey with me right from when it started. Some of them were there when I was imagining two hundred people in my room. When I hit two hundred subscribers, I thought, *Wow, what if all of those people were right here in my bedroom? They wouldn't all fit in here—that's a lot of people!* But amazingly, those two hundred people pushed a button to say they wanted me to be a part of their life.

When we're walking in downtown Pocatello or on the streets of LA, the guy who walks by and says, "Hi, Shay!" is in my house every day—because the people who watch me are part of our family. Men, women, kids, walk up and say, "I know this is weird but I feel like I know you so well. You have no idea who I am." But I do know who they are, because they know who I am, so we have a lot of stuff to talk about. They know my life. It's easy for them to say, "How's Babytard?" They know my children, my parents, my friends.

At first it was all so crazy and exciting that this was my career. But after a few years, the hype wears off and you have to ask yourself, *What is this about? Am I offering any kind of value to society?* I do, anyway. I want to know that it's not just about me posting cute videos of me and my family day in, day out. Plumbers help people by fixing their toilets, and construction workers help people by building houses and factories and offices. How am I helping people? The only way I know to answer that is to look at the comments, and they show that what we're doing is worth it. There are people who would pay a million dollars—or a hundred, or ten, or whatever they have—to be able to smile and feel better about themselves. The emails, the tweets, the comments, all the feedback we get from the people who watch tells us that we do offer a lot to people.

Our subscribers have choices. They don't have to watch us. They could be watching a reality show about a family that fights all the time and tears each other down. Instead, they choose to watch our family having a good time. It makes them smile.

A lot of people like to smile, it turns out. It's a thing that's catching on. Try it.

Day 15

A World Without Doughnuts

I **WAS BACK IN** LA yesterday to do a shoot in Santa Clarita and I stopped at a gas station to fill up. I was thinking, *A Coke sounds so good right now.* I wanted a Coke so bad. *You should have one,* my mind was saying. I went to order the Coke, and it was so hard to hold back—but then the act of resistance felt so good.

I started thinking about all the Cokes I've had in my life. Normally, I would buy that Coke at the gas station, which is about two hundred and fifty calories. Then when we'd go out to eat, I'd have at least two or three Cokes—you know, to help the food slide down. That's four or five hundred calories, a large part of it made up of sugar and chemicals. In a week, I'd ingest a couple thousand calories in Coke alone.

This is what I mean by how small decisions can make a big difference. Most people like to eat lunch, right? I love it! Let's say that you're a person who eats lunch every day. Let's say that you also like Coke and you have a twelve-ounce can of it with your lunch every day. Just a twelve-ounce can (don't get me started on those sixty-ounce buckets of diabetes that flow like a fountain from the nearest gas station) contains around 130 calories, and there are about 3,500 calories in one pound of fat.

Do the math with me here: your tiny twelve-ounce can of Coke you have for lunch every day, multiplied by the days in the year, makes you almost fourteen pounds fatter by the end of the year. The sums look like this:

130 calories x 365 days = 47,450 calories

Divided by the number of calories in a single pound of fat:

47,450/3,500=13.557 pounds of fat

Imagine what that one can of Coke per day does to you over five years. In fact, I'll help you out with the math again—that's 67.7 pounds of Coca-Cola Classic hanging around your forty-eight-inch waist. Try bending over to tie your shoes after gaining sixty-seven pounds of fat. It's hard to breathe! Do you really like Coke that much?

As I walked out of the gas station with no Coke in my hand, I also started thinking about all the doughnuts I've had in my life. And I asked myself, *What if I could take every doughnut I'd ever eaten and remove all of those doughnuts from my dietary equation?* You know what I'm saying? What would my body look like right now if I had never in my whole life consumed a doughnut? I've probably eaten a couple hundred doughnuts over the span of my life so far—heck, if I ate one a month from age ten to the present, that would be three hundred doughnuts right there. A chocolate-frosted doughnut has around two hundred and seventy calories, so that makes for a grand total of eighty-one thousand calories. Whoa boy.

The small things matter—they honestly do. Just start saying that and believing it. The little thoughts and decisions you make every single day are slowly and almost imperceptibly making you either better or worse. This is something that took me almost thirty-four years and plenty of struggle to truly understand. Because knowing is only half the battle. Heck, it's really only, like, 10 percent of the battle. The other 90 percent is in the action—the doing of the thing, if you will. Knowing is nothing without action.

This is my goal for this book and this summer, as I work with my son Gavin to teach him to make wise choices that will bring him health, strength, and happiness.

The small things add up when you consider what you consume day-in day-out, or even month-in month-out. Luckily, the same is true of exercise, and Gavin and I are discovering that we can make our day more energetic by sneaking little pieces of activity into the cracks. We're working on finding little opportunities throughout the day to get active. For instance, one of Gavin's chores is taking out the trash, and he's found a way to make that chore part of his exercise.

GAVIN: The trash cans are at the very bottom of our driveway and we have a big Dumpster right at the top. So I bicep curl the trash bags as I walk all the way up the hill.

SHAY: That's a pretty good workout right there.

Our bodies were meant to work. If we were living thousands of years ago, from the moment we woke up we would be active about getting the food we need to survive. I've got a watermelon sitting here on the bench beside me as I write, and back then, you would have had to go out and cut that melon off the vine in order to eat it. Just think about all the work it took to get different kinds of food, even if it wasn't the obvious activity of running down a beast and killing it. These days our lives are so easy in comparison, but we have the same need to generate energy. If you see me at the airport, you'll see me taking the stairs instead of the escalator. I want to take any opportunity to multitask: to get where I need to go, and burn extra energy along the way.

For me, a trip to Disneyland is a big workout day. When we go there, I know it's going to be exhausting with five kids—all that walking and standing in lines and carrying tired kids later in the day. From the moment I wake up, I make sure to drink plenty of water, do lots of stretching, and wear good shoes for what is essentially a full day of exercise. I don't think, *This is hot and annoying and hard work*; I think of it as a big training day for me. Disneyland is the equivalent of going on a big twenty-mile run because you're walking so far and carrying kids all day, and I love it. I'm feeling my biceps and trying to get a good workout. Sometimes you have to change your perspective and see exercise as a way to use your body positively.

The other great thing about a Disneyland workout day is you get to work out and eat churros at the same time. Nothing could be better than that. I'm not eating churros right now, of course. They do have a teensy amount of sugar in them, apparently. What I *am* doing is eating lots of small meals throughout the day. If your body thinks you're withholding food, it goes into starvation mode. *Hold up, Beardy McBeardson!* it says. *You're not going to feed me? Well, then I'm keeping this fat—I'm gonna hold on to it tightly, and I'm not letting go.* In starvation mode, your body stores the fat and starts burning muscle instead. And you don't want that because you want to be buff, right?

But if you keep eating small meals every couple of hours throughout the day, your body thinks, *This is fine, we keep getting food in here, everything is good.* Especially if you're eating a lot of fruits and vegetables, you really can eat as much of that as you want. You just need to be careful with the nuts; you can't go eating a pound of cashews. In fact, some people say you shouldn't eat nuts, but there's such a thing as good fat. Nuts are packed full of unsaturated fat, which helps to lower your cholesterol, so it's extra good for your heart.

Keep eating, keep snacking, and remember the incidental exercise. Do those bicep curls when you take out the trash—it's going to make trash time feel like it really means something.

Day 16

Here Comes the Asphalt Pie

There have definitely been times when I've really wanted something that's not healthy and we've been able to talk each other through it. The other night I was eating homemade pizza, and we talked about how it's not healthy to eat another slice just because we want it.

Last night, Gavin and I were so, so tempted to have a cheat day. We had a guest visiting, so we all headed to one of our favorite local restaurants called Wingers. On their dessert menu they have this most delicious, amazing, wicked creation called asphalt pie. It's essentially a giant slab of peppermint ice cream studded with chocolate chips, and underneath it all is a glorious, crunchy Oreo crust. It doesn't stop there, though: right on top there's a mound of whipped cream, with beautiful caramel drizzled all over the whole monumental pile of goodness.

You know why they call it asphalt pie? Because it's not your ass's fault that it gets so big when you eat it.

Our family loves it, so out comes this big plate of calorific destruction with ten spoons around it. Colette and the girls and our guests grab their spoons and dig in, and Gavin and I just look at each other. I can see we're both thinking the same thing. And I said to him, "Dude, what if we just had one cheat day?"

But we resisted and stayed strong. We just chewed spoons while we watched our family demolish that asphalt pie.

Food is a great joy for us: it's about pleasure and adventure and celebration. Over the past few years, we've had the good fortune to travel to some cool places and visit some outstanding restaurants. Gavin will try anything: escargot, chicken feet—you name it, he'll try it. He loves to cook and he's a great cook, too. I don't want to take that pleasure away from him, but we both need to change the associations whenever we put something in our mouth, so that "sweet" doesn't necessarily equate to "treat."

Back when I was running fifteen, twenty miles a day training for marathons, I felt like I could eat whatever I wanted. Any fuel I put in just got burned up and turned into energy. When I ran the St. George Marathon in Utah—one of the most beautiful anywhere, and mostly downhill and super fast—I ate vegan, which was such an epiphany for me. I felt clean and steady and confident and clear. *Why would I ever not do this?* I thought at the time. But somehow we slip. You indulge in something like a double bacon cheeseburger or a giant-size Coke, and you think, *Oh, it doesn't matter if I have just one.* But it does. It really does. It's a testament to the fact that small things matter. Those tiny things, those single choices, make a big difference.

The things we do make up who we are. Even if you eat junk food "just once," it means you have done it once and you will do it again. I went from that moment of feeling so good, so healthy, exercising and eating clean and thinking, *Why would I ever not do this?* to a year later thinking, *Oh crap, I'm forty pounds overweight.*

Let's say you go on vacation for a week. You've worked hard all year and you deserve that vacation, but if you're like most of us, you don't work out while you are on vacation; you relax and eat out and indulge yourself. Maybe you gain five pounds, then you go home and you don't feel like working out. Three months slip by, and then all of a sudden you can't breathe when you bend down to tie your shoes.

Even so, you keep lying to yourself: *I'm still in shape, I work out.* Another three months slide by and you think, *Wait a minute, I haven't worked out in how long?* If you're honest, you will tell yourself, *No, I am not in shape anymore.*

Maybe you finally realize how much things have changed when you want to do something energetic. You're playing soccer with your kids or throwing a football around with your buddies, and you're sucking wind and feeling like crap. *Man, what happened?* you think. *How did I get back to this?*

You have to pull yourself out of the spiral. The scary thing is, for a lot of people, that can be a twenty-year descent. Whoops, two decades just slipped by. Then it seems insurmountable to turn your health and your habits around. Or maybe just five years slip by and you have a couple of kids, and your whole lifestyle changes. It feels so hard, but you have to start with that first step, the one little thing that creates change and gets you to where you're going.

Sure, it's easy to say, *I'm just coasting, just staying the same.* But every single day, you're getting a little worse or a little better. There is no option to just chill for a while. It's a battle every day: with sugar, with exercise, with every decision, no matter how small. Either you're going this way or you're going that way. There is really no coasting.

Think about the difference between eating an apple and munching on a candy bar. It's as if you're at a point of homeostasis and a candy bar will pull you down, but an apple will pull you up. Those are the opportunity costs, the consequences of choosing this over that. Every time we're putting something in our mouth, those consequences need to be in our minds.

Apple = good.

Banana = good.

Water = good.

Saying no to sugar and processed foods is tough at first. As a society, we are so addicted. It's in all of our foods: our sauces, our packaged goods, our bottled drinks, our bread. Salt and sugar are both addictive, and therefore they sell, so the food companies decide, *Let's put those in whatever we're making.* Here's what my grandfather used to say: companies will spend millions of dollars on marketing a new product, coming up with a fancy new bottle and a new label. But when Johnny from product development asks, *Well, what are we going to put in it?* the CEO replies, *The same crap we always put in it, Johnny.*

It's hard to not take those delicious, fast highs because they're so easy, they're cheap, they're easy to grab, they're fun-looking. The packaging, the texture—it's all part of this seduction that's ultimately killing us. Salt and sugar are two substances our body craves, and we have to say no to them. As we do that more and more and eat natural foods and drink water, we achieve an equilibrium so we don't have those spikes and urges.

I feel like it gets easier the longer you go. I picked up the girls from a friend's place the other day, and they all had Skittles. I love Skittles: they're chewy, they're fruity, they're candy. That's my favorite type of sugar. I thought about it for a brief second, how nice it would be to have a few Skittles, and then I thought, *No, I'm not doing that right now.* It was that easy. I didn't dwell on it. I felt that initial craving and imagined what those Skittles would taste like in my mouth, but because I'm getting used to saying no to sugar, I was over it in seconds. Before, in the first week, I would've kept thinking about it and starting to justify maybe having one. Now that Gavin and I have been off candy for two weeks I'm used to that decision. It's not as difficult. I think that's true for all difficult decisions.

Sure, there are times I'm tempted to cheat. Late at night, when everyone else is in bed asleep, I open the fridge and have a staring contest with a half-eaten, week-old piece of birthday cake.

If it wasn't Gavin and me doing this challenge together, I definitely would have cheated. But the better part of my brain, the part that has the good ideas and the higher impulses, tells me, *My little boy believes in me. Gavin would be so disappointed.* For me as a father, I can't see how I could cheat when Gavin is doing so well. I feel so committed to him, and I hope he feels the same way. I'm also committed to myself, but there's definitely something to be said about being in a partnership and feeling that you don't want to let the other person down because you know that they're under the same weight that you are. You want to be strong for them because they're being strong, so it helps you to be stronger in a moment when you feel weak. Even if that's the one last thing that keeps you from breaking, it's worth it.

We've been having lots of visitors over throughout the summer, so there's been plenty of eating out and lots of pizza; it's one of those things that's so easy to make for a crowd. The other easy thing about pizza is eating too much of it! It's okay to have a slice or two occasionally, but there comes that point where you want another slice and you need to slow down. It tastes so good and you don't really need more, but you want to eat more.

Gavin and I have eaten pizza with our friends during this challenge. It may not seem like the healthiest choice, but the pizza we're eating is homemade, topped with plenty of fresh vegetables, and not processed, so we feel like we are getting more nutrients than if we ordered a standard pizza from Domino's. The other night, Gavin ate a slice, but I could see he was struggling with wanting another slice, so I said to him, "If you're full, stop."

Here's the thing about messing up, though. If you mess up, don't quit. If you say, "I can't stand it, I have to have some Doritos!" and you throw down one of those family-size bags of Doritos, don't feel like you have to give up because it's too hard and you've failed in that moment. Just get back on track, you know what I'm saying? Don't give up if you mess up. My good friend Brett Lemick once told me an analogy that went something like this: Don't give up on a healthy lifestyle just beause you have one bad day. When you get a flat tire, you don't get out of your car and stab the other three tires. You fix the flat tire, turn up the music, and keep driving!

Day 17

Honor and Cupcakes

One thing that kind of inspired me and my dad to write this book was an event that happened during my one-year sugar bet. It happened at my old school in LA. It was someone's birthday, and so of course they brought cupcakes in for a treat. This one kid noticed I didn't get a cupcake, so he came over and said, "Do you want a cupcake?" I said, "No thank you." Then he asked me why I didn't want one and I told him about my sugar bet. Then he said, "Well, dude, you can just eat a cupcake and not tell your

parents." I told him that I didn't want
to lie to my parents.

When Gavin came home and told me that story, I was so proud of him. This kid was trying to get him to eat a cupcake, but Gavin stood up to him. He told the other kid no, and on top of that, he explained that he didn't want to lie to his parents. That's an awesome story.

A lot of things happened in that situation. Gavin had to stand up to peer pressure, and he had to be able to say no to one of his classmates, which is not easy, especially at a young age like that. Then he had to say no to something that he probably really wanted. That's when your sense of honor shows itself, and that's when you become the kind of person that other people respect: someone with integrity.

Temptation comes from those little voices inside your head and from the voices outside your head as well: your best friends, your siblings, your colleagues. When you choose to live differently from your version of "the norm"—whether that means not eating fast food or sugary treats, or not drinking alcohol—people around you will try to persuade you to get back on their bandwagon. For kids and adults alike, it takes character to withstand that pressure. It's easy to fall for the easy.

But doing something that's easy won't give you any glory. There's no virtue in mediocrity. Doing hard things is valuable, right? By "hard things" I'm talking about everyday temptations, like saying no to a cupcake, or steering your shopping cart past the chips in the supermarket, or choosing a salad when your friends are ordering burgers.

When you're tempted to go with the flow and eat those fries or that candy bar or that pastry that's holding you back from being healthy, it's necessary to ask yourself, *Is it worth it?* A lot of times, you don't even consciously enjoy the thing you're eating; you're just throwing it into your mouth while you look at your phone.

Maybe if we ate our food with a little bit of self-awareness instead of shoveling it into our faces while we're scrolling through our Facebook timelines, we wouldn't eat as much. A lot of times, we're consuming our food like a drug. We're not even enjoying the experience of it, we're just getting it into our bodies as fast as possible so we can feel the effect. That's dangerous, and it's not why we eat. Chew, and slow down. Slowly take a bite and chew it, and enjoy the aroma and the flavor and the feel of it in your mouth.

Every time you put something into your mouth, ask yourself, *Is this helping the machine that's keeping me alive?* And if the answer is no, well, sometimes that's okay, but you then have to ask yourself, *How often am I going to allow myself to put something in that doesn't help the inside of me?* Weigh the opportunity cost. Is it worth the five minutes of pleasure if it means you can't run fast, sleep as well, or feel comfortable in your own body? All the consequences that come with putting this thing in your mouth—are they worth it? You've got to weigh those ideas in your mind and try to keep everything in the balance. Maybe you'll decide, *Eh, it's not worth it. I'll just have an apple instead.*

Here's the thing: every time you go through that process of weighing the costs and benefits and choosing the more difficult option, you're building exactly the set of muscles that will help you win your healthy living challenge. I'm not talking about your quads, your glutes or your abs (though who doesn't want a great six-pack?). I'm talking about your character. You can literally choose pretty much any weight-loss program and it will work if you stick to it. But once it's over, chances are you'll go back to the same old habits that made your belt tight in the first place.

I'm not going to say losing weight is easy. But compared to keeping the weight off long-term, losing weight in the short term is as easy as falling off a log. The real struggle lies in those months and years after you reach your goal, when cinnamon rolls and giant cups of soda dance before your eyes every time you go to the movies, the mall, or the gas station. If you look outside of yourself, you'll be tempted. Even if you rely on external resources, like diet maintenance programs and gym memberships, you're more likely to fail than to succeed if you don't maintain awareness.

Oh Shay, I hear you say, *that's such a downer. We might as well all give up now and go eat ice-cream sundaes.* Hold on—there is one thing that will make all the difference in the world, and that is character. It's character that made Gavin turn down that cupcake, and it's character that will help you stick to your healthy-living principles, too. Here are just a few of the qualities you might already have that you can draw on:

Perseverance—same as when you stuck with that job you hated, you can stick with eating salad for lunch (you'll love it one day!).

Self-regulation—just like when you held back from telling your mom how much you hate the new paint color she's chosen for the house, you can hold back from running to the cupboard for comfort when you're angry or sad.

Zeal—just like revving up your daughter's softball team before a

big game, you can pump yourself up about going for a run in
the morning.

Kindness (to yourself)—if you can encourage your best friend
    when he or she is feeling bummed, you can do the same for
    yourself when you fall off your diet.

You have some of these strengths already, and you can work on the
areas where you know you're weak. Just by being aware that character
is the key to your success, you're already making a start.

We're talking about life lessons here. This is a weight-loss book,
but the choices we make with food, the way we react to everyday
stimuli—it's all the same. What kind of person are you? Are you glut-
tonous? Do you do everything to excess? The goal in this life is to chip
away at those rough edges of our personality so that we can find that
well-rounded, best-possible person within.

Some people might say, *Just be who you are, why try to change
yourself?* But is it really okay to be who you are if you're bitter, resent-
ful, envious, or selfish? I don't think so. I think if you're a selfish jerk,
you should try to change that about yourself.

Character strengths are what make any exercise regimen and diet
plan work: without prudence and self-restraint and determination,
nothing can change. With them, everything is possible.

Day 18

Big Shirts and Six-Packs

Today my dad asked me, "How do you feel when you go shopping for clothes? What goes through your mind?" Sometimes I find a shirt that's awesome! But then I put it on and look in the mirror and think, I don't like the way this shirt fits on me. And so I put it back-it sounds stupid, I know, but I don't want my friends or somebody to tell me that I'm fat. Sometimes I think I should get a bigger size so I can't see my stomach poking through the shirt. But I've found out that the bigger size kind of makes me look fatter. When I played soccer, I had a really small jersey, and yesterday I saw myself on some of the vlogs and thought, I don't look so bad after all. So yeah, I guess I'm just very self-conscious.

SHAY: So we were watching a video of you playing soccer yesterday, and you were thinking maybe your jersey was too tight.

GAVIN: I don't want my shirts to be tight because then my stomach hangs out. That's why I like big shirts.

SHAY: But when we were watching that soccer video, you said, "I don't look so bad." Has that opened your eyes—that maybe you don't look as big as you thought you did?

GAVIN: Yeah, kind of.

SHAY: Sometimes a big shirt can make you look bigger. You don't want a skin-tight one, sure, but I don't think you need to wear shirts as big as you do. Maybe you feel a little bit self-conscious, but once you saw yourself active in that soccer video you thought, *No, I look pretty good.* Dude, as we keep biking and playing soccer for our thirty minutes a day, you're going to start seeing a difference. There'll be a big difference in your performance on the field, too. If you get that coat of a few extra pounds off, you're going to be able to run a lot faster. You could see in that video that you were full stride on some of those goals and getting distance on those kids. One day you're going to be even more agile.

By the end of this challenge, you'll be heading into middle

school. We'll be doing some school shopping and that's going to feel sweet. You won't have to get the big sizes, and your clothes will feel good to wear. That's a big part of feeling good about yourself—feeling comfortable in your clothes. Going into middle school, you're going to be with some older kids and you want to feel confident, right?

GAVIN: I can imagine myself going in to middle school with a six-pack.

SHAY: You want to be that ripped? Well, we better get to work then, bro. Give me ten push-ups right now. I've never had a six-pack. I don't know if our body types allow for it. Getting a six-pack is tough, but through this summer, you're definitely going to see a big difference. I think that's going to be exciting. We'll hit it hard and then you'll feel good about yourself when you go back to school. That's a big deal; you want to be able to walk through those doors on that first day with a bit of swagger and say, "What's up, ladies!" That's not all that matters though, Gavin—why do you always turn every conversation to the ladies?

GAVIN: I think that was you, Dad.

SHAY: That's true. But now that I think about it, I had the opposite problem from you. When I was fat, I didn't want to let myself go above the size that I had always been. There's a great moment in a *Seinfeld* episode when Jerry gets caught marking out the size 32 on the waistband of his Levi's so it looks like he's still wearing size 31 jeans. I was like that when I was getting bigger. I just couldn't abide the idea that I was no longer a size so-and-so.

I can be a tougher critic of myself than anyone else on Earth. That's the other side of denial—that intense sense of self-consciousness, like everyone is checking you out and finds you lacking in some crucial way. We all do it, don't we?

Being so self-critical can really be a bummer; on the flip side, though, it can really give you a push when you see old photos of yourself looking good. Just the other day I was looking at some pictures of me when I was in better shape, and I want to look like that again! In those photos I was wearing a shirt that used to be one of my favorites, and I still have it scrunched up at the back of my closet. I know it won't fit me right now, but I love that shirt and I want to wear that shirt again. So maybe at the end of this challenge I'm going to take that shirt and put it on, without even having to stretch it on a chair! Man, how good does it feel to be able to put a shirt on and not feel like it's adhering to your skin and stretching out against your gut? That is such a good feeling, to check yourself out in the mirror and think, *Oh, now that looks pretty good.*

There are two other great ways to motivate yourself that I want to mention here, too. I've said it before but it's worth saying again: don't weigh yourself every day. It gets discouraging, trust me. If you're thinking, *I've gone for a day eating fruits and vegetables and being healthy—I'm going to hop on the scale,* and then you find you've only lost half a pound or none at all, that's going to be disheartening. Your weight doesn't matter right now; what matters is making those healthy decisions and making those your new habits.

The other way to motivate yourself is by reading books about healthy food and exercise. That totally helps because you learn as you go. You know I love *Fit for Life,* and if you read something like that, you could learn about how some food is toxic or useless to your body, which really helps you to stay away from those things.

Colette and I went to the movies the other night. If you're like us, you love smuggling treats and candy into the theater. I snuck in blueberries, cashews, and carrots, and when I pulled them out afterward, they looked kind of gross because they had all mashed together in my pocket. But anyway, it meant I could eat fresh snacks throughout the movie, which was good—better than popcorn. Movies were never as good to me without an enormous bucket of buttered popcorn, a giant Coke, and a huge bag of Twizzlers. But those are all for my taste buds; my body can't actually use those things for energy. The one thousand calories I used to consume during a movie were literally for taste alone. They're not going to help my body in any way, shape, or form. Just like we talked about a few days back, when you put those boxes in your body, some are easier to break down than others. When you're eating gummy bears, your body is thinking, *I can't do anything with this.* There's no nutritional value, they're just pieces of plastic.

If you're getting some good information about this and starting to feel good about what you're putting into your body and how you're using it to be active, that's when you can really set things to rights. You can tell your body: *No, adipose tissue, you will not envelop my belly, cause my pants to be tight around my waist area, and make my belt protrude into the lower area of my belly button until it hurts and I can't bend over.*

It's time to take a stand!

Day 19

The Motivation Cycle

SHAY: I think you're looking thinner. How do you feel? Do you feel different?

GAVIN: I feel good. I've lost seven pounds.

SHAY: Dude, have you been weighing yourself?

GAVIN: Well, just today.

SHAY: How much did you weigh before?

GAVIN: [silence]

SHAY: Are you embarrassed to say? That's okay. But do you *feel* like you've lost seven pounds?

GAVIN: Yeah.

SHAY: Then that's what matters.

The numbers don't mean much. I could weigh 180 pounds and be a super-fit dude who works out every day and eats healthy. Or I could weigh 180 pounds and have zero aerobic fitness, blood pressure through the roof, smoking a pack a day. Same number, but polar opposite in terms of every health indicator you can imagine.

The trouble with body weight is, it doesn't tell us what that weight is made of. An elite athlete could have very little body fat but weigh the same as a heavier person because a pound of muscle takes up less space than a pound of fat. Similarly, you could have a "skinny" fat person who doesn't weigh much but has very little muscle mass, high blood pressure, and high cholesterol.

I haven't been weighing myself since we started this, but I can feel I've lost some weight over the past few days. Thing is, I'm not feeling all that pumped about it because it wasn't a result of living an awesome lifestyle—it was because I've had a stomach flu. It's not great to lose ten pounds because you've been pooping and vomiting for days. Gavin and I had been down in LA and we were due to fly back to Idaho, but I didn't know if I could make it. We almost cancelled our flight, but I just needed to get back home. So I took a bunch of Advil and we went for it. Then when I got home, I lay in bed for four days, and everyone told me I looked like I had lost a ton of weight.

But I feel good now. I've got my energy and strength back. I've been going to CrossFit, but I haven't wanted to drag Gavin along with me during that challenge. I wanted him to build his own routine. I wanted him to know that even if Dad's not here, he has everything he needs to work out and get his heartbeat going. The day before yesterday and today, he did three miles on the treadmill while I went to CrossFit. (He slacked off yesterday, but I don't want to give him a hard time about it. This is what progress looks like.)

So there is healthy weight loss and unhealthy weight loss; a low number isn't necessarily a good thing. Yet people load that little number up with so much meaning. We get to comparing ourselves, and before you know it, a little set of blinking red numbers on a device sitting on our bathroom floor has become something bigger. Something to be proud or ashamed of.

I do use weight as one concrete way to measure the changes in my body and something to keep me focused, especially when we're doing a thirty-day challenge like this. Most of all, though, I want to feel better.

One of the reasons we moved back to Idaho after being in Los Angeles for five years was so our kids could experience the same carefree summers Colette and I enjoyed as kids. We moved to LA to start a YouTube business with some other YouTube friends, which became Maker Studios, and during that time we uploaded five years of daily vlogs to our YouTube channel, Shaytards. Over five years and almost two thousand videos later, we grew an audience of over two million subscribers. We showed our audience everything: dancing, shouting, laughing, crying, two of our babies being born, our beloved dog Malachi reaching the end of his life. But in LA, I could never let my kids just run out in the front yard and down to their friend's house on the corner to build a rope swing over the gully. I couldn't—that stuff is just too dangerous in a big city. What if a crazy person shot them or something? My brother Casey and I had such an active childhood, and we were always outdoors. We played soccer, basketball, and baseball, and we loved to skateboard and rollerblade and ski. I wanted my kids to experience the fun and freedom I had growing up, so we came back to Idaho and bought a big chunk of land—big enough to build a soccer field on, which is what we're doing right now. Since soccer is

Gavin's passion, he's pretty excited about that. Once the field is ready, we'll both be out there quite a bit.

SHAY: I think you'll see an improvement in your game, Gavin. Once you start shedding some of those pounds, you'll be able to do more of those neat moves and run faster to the ball. Then you'll become better at soccer, which will motivate you to want to lose more weight and stay healthy, and once you do that some more, you'll get into what's called the motivation cycle. When you work hard at something that's tough, you see a few results, and those results motivate you. It gives you more gas to keep pushing. So you push a little bit harder, and then because you pushed harder, guess what happens.

GAVIN: You're really healthy, and you see more results?

SHAY: And when you see more results, how do you feel?

GAVIN: More motivated.

SHAY: And if you're more motivated, what do you do?

GAVIN: You keep going.

SHAY: And then when you work harder, what do you see?

GAVIN: More results.

SHAY: And when you see more results, how do you feel?

GAVIN: Motivated.

SHAY: And when you feel motivated, what do you do?

GAVIN: Work harder?

SHAY: And when you work harder, what do you see?

GAVIN: Results.

SHAY: Results! And when you . . . you see? It's this cycle. So we've got to push ourselves until we see results, and when we see those results, we've got to celebrate those results. You're looking good, you're feeling good, you say, "Awesome job! Let's work harder and keep pushing." But it's hard to get that cycle started, right? It's like getting a train going, getting those big iron wheels slowly starting up. But once they start, it's exciting—*Yeah, yeah, we're seeing it, it's working! It's working! Whooo, we're ripped!* And that's when it gets easier and easier.

Starting that cycle is the hard part, but we're in week three now, so we're rolling. Let's not give up, let's keep going. Let's hit those workouts every day and let's drink our water. We're going to see more results and we'll get into that motivation cycle. It will just get easier and easier and easier.

Day 20

Fatherhood

YESTERDAY WAS FATHER'S DAY, and in my twelve years of being a dad, it was probably the very best Father's Day I've ever had. I got a motorcycle, which is one of the coolest presents I've ever received. (I'll wear a helmet all the time, I promise.) I had such a great time hanging out with my own dad and being with my kids and my mom and my family. That's what living is all about: just being with them.

When Gavin was just a baby, I worked such long hours during the week that I hardly saw him or Colette. When you're putting that much time into a job during the weekly Monday to Friday grind, you begin to really, really love the weekends. After all, what was the point of working so hard if I couldn't spend time with the people I loved the most?

Once we could afford a few nice things, we started to eat out more often. Friday and Saturday nights became our escape from the mundane world and our daily schedules, and our favorite was steak and Malibu chicken at Sizzler. Does Sizzler also have an all-you-can-eat ice-cream bar? *Yes!* Did we eat heaps of it and feed that ice cream to our adorable new baby? *Yes!* Then of course after dinner, it was movie night! We had a little money, but not enough to buy movie theater candy, so we would sneak in piles of candy we bought from the dollar store, stashed into our bags.

It became our ritual. *Hate your life and work all week so you can party on the weekend with delicious food!* At first I still felt like the healthy, wrestle-a-bear-to-the-ground kind of dude I always had been, but over those first few years of marriage, little by little, some differences started to show. My jeans started to shrink, my belts got shorter, my toes farther from my head. At least that's how it felt, because it became harder to pull my jeans up, harder to buckle my belt through the hole I usually used, harder to reach down to my feet to pull on my shoes. Our favorite rituals were setting me on a conveyor belt—not a path; that would have required too much walking—to packing on more weight.

I wasn't fat, exactly—I just had a little extra Shay on me.

And since our way of getting happy on the weekends involved indulging in food, I reasoned that any time our baby boy was unsettled or crying, it was nothing a nice big bottle of cow's milk wouldn't cure. Later on, it became a cracker, or a cookie, or a French fry, but it was always food or drink that was the solution, the way of making everything seem better.

The other thing about being a dad is, you have to take responsibility. And I have to face up to the fact that in those early years of Gavin's life, we had a lot of fun but we also didn't lead the healthiest of existences. Through the choices I made then, I set my son and myself in a particular direction, and since then it has been difficult to turn around and make healthy food choices, to choose water over pop, and to make exercise a basic part of our everyday life. Those are the things I want to change now.

Here's the thing, though: it's because I'm a father that this healthy living challenge we're doing means more than anything to me. The reason I'm doing this with Gavin is that I want to live longer, so I can have more experiences with my family and strengthen our relationships with each other. That's our answer to the "why" question: because our family relationship is the most important thing.

Part of what I believe is that everybody on this earth lived with God before we were born. We were all brothers and sisters there, part of a large family of people. Now we're all here on earth to gain a physical body and to learn from our experiences, no matter our country of origin, religion, race, color, or beard.

That's why I lost weight in the first place. When I was at my heaviest, I was almost three hundred pounds and eating so unhealthily that if I played with my kids I would get winded after just a couple of minutes. I couldn't live the life I wanted to live with my wife and children. I was motivated to lose weight because I didn't want to die before I had truly *experienced* the experiences I was placed on this earth to have.

I've put too much into these relationships for them to end at mortality, though. I also believe that we live after this life and that we will live together as a family forever. I don't believe that we're just married until "death do us part"; marriage is eternal. But I don't want to tell you what to believe. The whole point is that you need to ask these questions for yourself. *What do I believe? What am I trying to get out of this life? Am I just destined to become worm food?* For me, I believe that I've worked too hard on my relationship with this hot chick I'm married to. I don't want to become worm food too soon.

This is why health matters beyond the here and now. We've had some early deaths in my family, and if I die when my grandpa died, that means I only have another twenty years left. I want to reverse that. I want more time to be a dad. And I want many, many more Father's Days.

Day 21

Powering Up

> I've learned that when I'm hungry, I'm not always actually hungry, I'm just thirsty, and usually I haven't been drinking enough water that day. But since we began this challenge, I've been motivated by the competition, so it made me want to drink more water than my dad, which is helping me meet our goal.

Finally! We've done really well with the water aspect of the challenge this past week. We've been able to stay on top of our goal by carrying a gallon jug with us wherever we go, which has been great for staying hydrated but isn't always the most convenient. Yesterday I drank half of my jug, then went to the gym on my motorcycle and took the jug with me. As I was coming back from the gym, I went over a bump and half the jug spilled all over the back of my pants, and it looked like I peed myself. One minute I was riding my motorcycle, free as a bird, the next minute I was soaking wet. I turned around and the jug had a big hole in the bottom and was shooting water out. Not good.

There's no end to the things that people criticize me for. They could say that I'm fat, or they hate my beard, or I'm egotistical—wait, they *do* say all those things—but mostly, they choose to pick at the little things, including the way I've been drinking water for this challenge. When I vlogged that we had bought fourteen jugs of water, people said, *Shay, that's so wasteful—why didn't you just get one jug and refill it?* Even the checkout dude in the grocery store muttered something. I swear I heard, "It's called tap water."

It was interesting that people were upset about us buying the jugs, but here's the thing: staying hydrated is one of the body's biggest priorities. Some of us have access to drinkable tap water, but some of us don't. Some of us are sedentary for most of the day and can hit the sink or the water cooler over and over again, but some of us aren't. You have to figure out a way to make staying hydrated work for you. My feeling is, as long as Gavin and I recycle our containers—which we're doing—we can use the jugs as physical reminders to drink more water. Not everyone needs it, but for people like us, who struggle to remember to drink enough water, it has been helping a lot.

GAVIN: What I noticed about drinking more water is that I definitely sleep a lot better. Sometimes when I wake up, I don't feel very good. If I drink a lot of water and then go to the bathroom in the morning, it really helps me out.

SHAY: What do you mean? It helps you poop?

GAVIN: Ummm—yeah. It's like it cleans me out for the morning, and then I'm ready to go about my day.

SHAY: Totally agree. On the downside, the thing I've been noticing is that sometimes I drink from a jug in the morning, and then by around lunchtime I kind of forget about it. Then by four or five o'clock in the afternoon I get that feeling that I just need to eat something right then and there. I go into the kitchen thinking, *Oh, I'm so hungry.* Because we're doing the no-sugar thing, I pace around, opening cupboard doors, looking for something to eat. I'll have some baked chips and salsa, and then I'll snack on a couple of granola bars, but it won't do it for me. Finally, I'll think, *You know what? I'm thirsty.* Then I'll fill up a big glass of water, chug it, and take a deep breath and think, *Oh, wow. That's what I needed. I just needed some water.*

I'm starting to see water bottles as a power-up, like in a video game where you go a level up. You know those little sixteen-ounce water bottles, the smallest ones you can buy, the ones they hand out at kids' soccer games? Now imagine you're Mario and you're bouncing through level one and you see a mushroom—you want to get it because it makes you stronger, right? I see these little bottles of water the same way. It's hard to carry a gallon jug around every day—especially if you're riding a motorcycle—so any time I see a bottle of water, I grab it.

The other day we were camping and we were about to eat dinner when I saw two of those little water bottles in the back of my truck. To me, they were like water capsules: if I took them right then, before I ate, I'd feel way better. So I chugged those two little bottles and I *did* feel great. They say you're supposed to drink eight eight-ounce glasses of water a day (or thereabouts, but eight times eight is really easy to remember), so if I do that four times a day, that's my recommended daily water intake.

GAVIN: I've got another analogy. Water is like an avatar that blasts water out of his hands. He shoots all around in your body and the monsters on the wall scream, "Aaah!" Those fat monsters and sugar monsters fall off and get blown away.

SHAY: I love that! Another thing I've got going is that when we go out to dinner at a restaurant, we usually get water for the table first. I try to drink that first glass of water as fast as I can before the server comes back to take our appetizer order so she can see I'm thirsty. Even if I'm not, I force myself to chug a glass of water. My goal is to drink two glasses of water before our food shows up at the table. That way, I know for a fact that I'm only going to eat what I need; I won't end up eating unnecessary calories just because I'm trying to satiate myself when all I really am is dehydrated and maybe a little bit hungry.

When I'm not so determined about drinking the right amount of water, I eat double the portions that I probably would have otherwise, and on top of that I'm still dehydrated. I think we can save ourselves a little chub around the midsection just by drinking the right amount of water.

After the last few days, water has become like that level up in a video game. Now that I have this ally on my side and I've seen its benefits, I don't want to go without utilizing my secret weapon. Best of all, it's free and it's everywhere—in developed countries at least, which is a gift and a privilege in itself.

What are the things that have to go into our body for us to survive? Air is number one. None of us forget to breathe enough air, right? Nobody's going around saying, *Hey, be sure to breathe your ration of air today.* But the second most important thing is water. You can survive a lot longer without food than without water. It's a well-known fact that you could live for about three weeks if you didn't have any food—chubby guys like me, we could maybe live six weeks. Then I would eat Gavin after he died, so I'd probably hang on for six months. But you have to have water—you're going to die after about three days without water. You've got to have the wet stuff in you to get the oxygen moving around, to flush out the waste, to keep the organs working. Experts in survival call it the "rule of threes": three minutes without air, three days without water, three weeks without food.

Water gets overlooked because it's boring. There are no bubbles, there's no taste, it's not exciting. There are people who don't drink water except by accident, when they're brushing their teeth, or when the ice melts in their forty-ounce thirst buster. Their poor bodies. While we've been drinking our gallons a day, our skin has been cleaner, I can see Gavin looking trimmer, and we've been sleeping better. I wake up with the sun now.

And if you stay hydrated, you don't wake up with that gross, nasty morning mouth. You know when you wake up and you feel like you need to hock a loogie but your throat is too clogged up to do it? That's all the chemicals your body tried to get rid of throughout the night. When you drink enough water, you don't get that. Not as bad, anyway.

Nothing gives me more of a kick than seeing Emmi and Brock and the other kids joining in on some of our healthy living challenge. The water jug thing especially caught on with them. We bought Brock a little one-liter water jug, and pretty soon all of the Butlers were carrying their jugs around. It became a shared family habit. After a while, it got confusing as to who owned what jug, so we wrote our names on them. You could walk through the room where I'm sitting right now and pick up a half-dozen half-empty water jugs. If you didn't know what was going on, you would think we were kind of weird. Same as usual, really.

Day 22

Riding to Canada

When my dad decided to run a marathon, I thought it was crazy and cool at the same time. Crazy because it's hard to run a marathon and it would be his first one. But I figured it was pretty cool, too.

We're looking for more active things to do together, so I want to get Gavin a road bike. This morning we went for a ride together and that was cool, but he was on his mom's bike and it's a little big, so I want to get him a bike of his own. Once he gets used to the gears, we can cruise the roads maybe three times a week. That can be our goal for this weekend, to get him that bike. I've got to go to the bike shop on Saturday to pick up my bike—I dropped it off for a tune-up—so we'll get Gavin a bike, then we can start cruising these roads and drinking our water, just two healthy guys.

I owe bike riding a lot; it was really how I started to get active. At my heaviest, I was 280 pounds. We were living in LA at the time and I decided I was going to run the Los Angeles Marathon. I got it in my bones and was determined that I was going to do this thing because I had always said I wanted to run a marathon. Deep down, I thought it was crazy that anybody could run continuously without stopping for 26.2 miles. But as somebody who wants to do big, cool, and possibly crazy things, running a marathon was one of my life goals. I had talked about it forever, and I decided now was the time. But I was big, and I was so, so not in shape.

The very first run I went on was just around the block. My knee hurt, my ankle hurt, my side hurt. All of these pains were in the places you would expect pain, as well as less expected areas. I'm pretty sure I experienced some discomfort in my hair follicles. I was this big, jumbling tub of lard running down the street. If I could barely make it around the block because it hurt so much, I had no idea how I was going to run 26.2 miles.

Running even a mile was so agonizing, but I knew I could definitely ride a bike a couple of miles, so I figured I'd start biking. I got a red-and-white mountain bike and I started riding that instead of running. That first day I went for a three-mile bike ride. That was the beginning. After that, every day I would try to go a little bit farther. The next day I decided I was going five miles. I just kept going and going and going.

From where we lived in Venice, there's a path that goes up to Malibu, alongside the Pacific Ocean, and it has the most amazing views, with a beautiful breeze flowing in from the ocean. I would ride up this path a little farther every day, going a mile, two miles, three miles, then turn around. I never knew how far this path went up the coast, but in my mind I liked to imagine that it went all the way to Canada. I liked that idea, but I never knew because I couldn't make it to the end of the path; instead, I'd get tired and have to turn around for home.

On those first rides, I got such a kick out of going a little bit farther than I did the day before. As the days went by, I became intensely curious about where this path went. I could have looked it up on my GPS, but it became this little mystery: every day I ventured out on this bike path, but I didn't know where it went.

Eventually I worked up to eleven miles, then fifteen. Then I decided that the next day I was going to take some money with me, because even if I had to stop for lunch, I didn't care: I was just going to go as far as I could. I rode to the point I had reached the day before and then I kept going another mile, and another, and I made it to the very end of the trail, which is in Malibu. Not Canada, but that was fine. From where our house was to the end of the trail in Malibu, it was a twenty-mile bike ride. *Holy crap. I just rode my bike twenty miles!*

By the time I got up to the point of being able to do that, I had lost a good chunk of weight, probably thirty or forty pounds, and I was ready to start running and training for that marathon.

Around that time, too, Gavin and I started going on bike rides together. We even went on a seventeen-mile ride together along that same path.

GAVIN: Now that we're back in Idaho, we live up in the mountains, and riding here is a lot harder because of the elevation. There are a lot of hills, which makes it hard, but there's some downhill parts where you go past huge fields of flowers. It's really pretty.

SHAY: When we were coming up that hill this morning, we were saying how pretty it was, and the look on your face said, *Shut up about the flowers.* We live in a valley, so if you want to go out on your bike, either way involves going uphill. From the bottom of our driveway there's a huge uphill climb to the right, but if you go left, it's downhill for a little while, then uphill. And we're at a 6,500 feet elevation. So the roads are not easy for bike riding. It's hard, it's intense.

Looking back even further, it was actually a bike that gave me my first lesson in breaking bad habits, too, though not my own in this particular case. As you know, when I was nineteen years old, I left my home in Idaho to go to the West Indies on a two-year service mission for my church. I lived on the islands of Barbados and Trinidad, and I spent ten months in Guyana, on the northern tip of South America. I spent those two years helping the people of the Caribbean to overcome habits that controlled and sometimes dominated their lives. One man was struggling to quit smoking cigarettes. His wife and three grown-up children were worried about his health: his doctors had told him that if he didn't stop smoking and begin living a healthier lifestyle, he was dangerously at risk of a heart attack, and he had early signs of lung and throat cancer.

My mission companion and I were determined to help this man overcome this weakness. In our white shirts and ties, we would sit with him and have long talks about quitting. He *wanted* to quit smoking—he knew he had to quit if he wanted to hang around and see his grandchildren one day. In desperation, I went to a local pharmacy in Barbados and asked the pharmacist what kind of things a person who wanted to stop smoking should do.

"You have to replace the habit," the pharmacist told me. He explained that the simple habit of raising your hand to your face to smoke a cigarette becomes deeply ingrained if you do it hundreds of times each day, year after year. He suggested that we tweak the habit by replacing the cigarette with a sucker. The habit of raising your hand to your mouth stays intact, but the nicotine is gone. Of course he would have to be careful to brush his teeth more regularly, but at least he wouldn't be smoking anymore.

That sounded like a brilliant idea to me, so we got our friend a big bag of suckers and told him that every time he was tempted to smoke a cigarette, he had to grab a sucker instead. He tried it out for a few weeks and still couldn't quit. The suckers were helping, but he still had to have that morning cigarette right after waking up. It was almost impossible for him to start his day without at least one cigarette. He'd been doing it for over twenty years, and quitting one of the most addictive substances known to man was not going to be solved by a bag of suckers and two eager Mormons.

We didn't give up on him, though, and we suggested that he start going for morning bike rides right when he woke up. We even arranged to meet him on our missionary bicycles for the first few mornings. He loved it! He was the type of guy who liked to talk to everybody in the neighborhood, and so he loved that he had an excuse to ride past all of his favorite gossip spots.

Those rides were far from Tour de France training sessions, but he put in a few miles on his old beach cruiser. It was just the change he needed to break free of the deathly grip of nicotine.

It was so exciting for me! I was so proud of him, and at the same time, I was getting my first lesson in habits—how they form, and how to break them. I was starting to see that the small things matter. Each step, each mile on the bike, takes us closer to our goal.

Day 23

No Excuses

This whole thing is already tough, but it's tougher, I think, because I have an ingrown toenail that I just had fixed, so it hurts if I touch it against something. I have to keep doing saline baths for it and it's a real pain.

Right in the middle of our challenge, Gavin got an ingrown toenail treated, which is kind of painful. The doctor lifted the nail up and put some cotton under it to help the nail grow properly, and now Gavin has to soak his toe in a saline solution a couple of times a day. It's a distraction, but in life, there are always distractions and reasons to give up.

All of us have different crosses to bear, but I don't like making excuses. My battle is, I have a hugely addictive personality. I know it. That's just who I am. If I do something, I do it all the way, and that can be a problem for me in life. But I have to deal with it. I've tried to teach Gavin that we all have problems and setbacks. We're both lucky to have two legs; some people don't have legs at all, so shut up. Until you've lost an appendage, you don't have any room to complain. I really believe in that. I believe in mind over matter.

GAVIN: Hey, there's a kid who doesn't have any legs, but he's a top wrestler.

SHAY: That's a great example—yeah, we saw a video of this kid, Isaiah Bird, who is six years old and was born without legs. He lives in a shelter with his mom and his little brother, and he's the fiercest wrestler: he loves it, says he doesn't need any legs to wrestle. And remember Nick Vujicic, the guy with no arms or legs who surfs? He was born like that, too, and now he swims and surfs and is a motivational speaker. There are people out there like that who have figured out how to break through. We watched a movie about Nick Vujicic and we thought, *Good for him, that's so amazing.* And then, of course, we went back to going about our own lives with two arms and two legs; we didn't have to wake up the next morning with no appendages. We didn't have to figure out how to do all the crappy stuff, like how to wipe your butt—all the stuff we don't even have to think about. Those mundane tasks are huge chores for him.

I know you can change your body. I don't want to hear your excuse about how you have a bum knee or no time or a house full of screaming kids. Because for every one of those excuses, there's an example of someone who faces the exact same thing you're dealing with, who has found a way to overcome it to achieve a healthy body, regardless of their limitations.

Someone like Nick could think, *My life sucks. I have to deal with this every day and nobody appreciates that, nobody has it as tough as I do.* He could decide to get angry and be bitter toward the world. He could choose to have the attitude, *I hate everybody. I'm pissed off.* But he doesn't. He chooses to be happy, because it doesn't feel good to be mad. It doesn't feel good to be unhealthy, either. Ultimately, what we want is to feel good and be happy. I believe we're designed to be happy—I mean, maybe we're designed to exist for other reasons, too, but we might as well be happy while we're at it. Making wise, responsible choices ultimately brings long-term happiness.

One of the biggest barriers to happiness and to progress in leading a healthy lifestyle is procrastination. It's always easier to do something hard the next day, especially when something is bugging you, like an ingrown toenail. Gavin, what's your insight on that? How do you stop avoiding the things you have to do?

GAVIN: Sometimes I'll procrastinate on book reports. I'll do it at the last second, and then it's not as good as it would have been if I'd spent longer on it. Even though I don't want to do it, you have to say, *It's a big part of your grade, you just have to do it and get it over with.*

SHAY: So another way of saying that might be, *There's pain from not doing it.* Right? How do you feel when you're trying to finish it right before it's due—do you feel anxious?

GAVIN: If you know you should be working on it but you're not, you have that feeling inside that says, *I should be doing this right now.*

SHAY: That's what I'm saying. Sometimes you have to measure that and you have to ask yourself, *What is worth more to me: being able to relax and do whatever I want, or having that anxious feeling because I'm not doing what I have to do?*

There's a great saying that I learned from my dad's father. It goes, "Work will work when nothing else will work." Grandpa Eugene was a colonel in the Air Force, so he knew a thing or two about hard work. He grew up having nothing, part of the generation that suffered through the Depression. In that era, you had to make do. You didn't own all the stuff we possess today. You didn't have a blender or a microwave or a dishwasher. You were lucky if you had a leather belt to cook up for dinner. We can't imagine what they went through.

Grandpa Eugene used to tell us stories about how his mom would leave him and his little brother for a week at a time so she could go find work because his dad was gone. From a young age, the two boys would be in the house alone. They would go out and forage for roots and grasses and eat them because they had no food—nothing at all. They were literally dirt poor.

But Grandpa Eugene was the epitome of the classic American success story—someone who learned to pull himself up by his bootstraps. He came from a very meager, humble situation in life and joined the military; then eventually he became a philanthropist. In the later years of his life, he lived in a big house in Provo and helped out a number of kids from the community in various ways, like paying for their college tuition at Brigham Young University.

When you went to Grandpa's house, things were done a certain way. He had an acronym for everything. The dishwasher was the DW, the wastebasket was the WB. "Shay, Casey, you empty the WB yet?" Back when I was sixteen or seventeen, Casey and I even made a skit about this—maybe I should put it on YouTube. We had this big old VHS camcorder and we made a video of us making fun of our grandpa for his eccentricities. His enchiladas were so spicy, but if you thought the jalapeños were too much, he'd call you a "gringo." We did this scene where we poured gasoline on a burrito and set it on fire, then I brought the flaming plate to the table like I was Grandpa.

"Here's your enchilada, Casey."

"Grandpa, it looks a little spicy."

"Don't be a gringo!"

He was so funny in certain ways. But most of all, he was a people person. The expression "he never met a stranger" was so true of my grandpa. He could talk to and be friends with anybody, no matter what their background, age, or point of view was. I do think I get a lot of my personality from him, even though I didn't spend a ton of time with him. He was active duty and living in Utah when we lived here in Idaho, but he was at all of the seminal life events. When I went on my mission, baptisms, weddings—Grandpa Eugene was always there.

Grandpa Eugene passed in 2008, when I had only just started doing YouTube. It sucked when he died because I would have loved for him to influence my kids in certain ways, so I try to remind them of him. Ultimately, I've realized that that's who we are: we are who we came from. We are part of a family line. I wouldn't be here without my dad, and my dad wouldn't be here if it wasn't for Colonel Eugene Haynes Butler. That means a lot to me, so I think about things my grandpa said, and did, and I want to make him proud. Saying no to excuses is part of that.

Day 24

Saving the Human Race

GAVIN IS GETTING really athletic. We had a big basketball game the other day with a bunch of employees from my clothing line, Trixin, and Gavin loved it. He was guarding Aaron, our tech guy; Aaron is around twenty-one years old, but they were pretty evenly matched. It was a battle between the two of them, and Gavin made some good fouls on Aaron. I was impressed that he was getting so physical and being so aggressive.

GAVIN: There was one time I was bouncing it out on the perimeter, and Aaron was saying, "Maybe I should give you space to shoot." I told him, "I don't need space."

SHAY: Oh yeah, he was smack talking. I think you like some competition.

At first we were going to nine, win by two. Then the next game Gavin suggested, what if we went to fifteen? He wanted to up the ante and play longer. But we decided to go to nine, win by one. We didn't go easy on Gavin, either. He was double-dribbling and making some fouls, and we were on him for that. Once he said, "Don't go easy on me," I was really getting after him. "Gavin, pay attention, where are you throwing it?" We were tied nine-nine, right in the heat of the game, a next point wins type of situation, and Gavin tried to make this fancy behind-the-back pass to Derek. It got intercepted, so I told him, "Bro, get your head in the game!" We had just watched the NBA finals together, so we knew what it's like when the time is ticking down and you have to get a score. That feeling of, *It's nine-nine, and I know these are our friends and coworkers, but we want to kick their butt right now* is exciting and fun, and it makes you work harder. We were tired, but I could see Gavin wasn't thinking about taking a break. He was thinking about going harder. We won that next point.

That's why sports are great: they're exercise but they're fun. Back at the beginning of all this, Gavin and I decided we were going to have the funnest summer ever, and I didn't ever want the exercise to feel like work. Sports are a big part of that. Sports are exercise with a purpose, and sometimes with a team—what could be better? Sports aren't life, though. When I go to my eight-year-old nephew's baseball game and the parents and coaches are getting so intense about it—that sucks. Come on, this is a game someone invented—this isn't life or death. Sports are great to play, but not to take too seriously. I wish I was the same age as Gavin, and that I could play basketball with him but still have my same thirty-five-year-old brain. Then I would definitely get in his head. I would definitely beat him. Gavin is way bigger than I was at his age, though. I was short. Like, two feet tall.

When I was eleven, my brother Casey and I were into every sport, and because we were very close in age, we were seriously competitive. We grew up playing everything. I did wrestling, cross-country, and all the team sports, as well as skateboarding and skiing. I did every sport there was up until ninth grade; then when I was in high school I switched over to skiing and I would just ski all the time. A little later on, I also got more into extreme sports, like rock climbing. For a year and a half, I was an intense rock climber.

I loved being active. I got voted most daring in middle school. Back in the day, when I was in high school, I was doing double back-flips off bridges into rivers. I was an adrenaline junkie, and I still am. If I didn't have a family, I would be doing a lot of different things that I can't do now. I think about that from time to time. Only a couple of years ago, I did a video with Devin Graham, known as devinsuper-tramp on YouTube, where I did this flip off a three-hundred-foot rope swing. Now I'm a little bit older and I have another kid, and I think to myself, *I shouldn't do that stuff anymore. I could die.*

But then, sometime in my twenties, I got fat, and I just let my fat cells get carried away with themselves. I was going to school and I wasn't thinking about my body, I was only thinking about trying to make money to provide for my family.

GAVIN: Maybe you were in a slump. Some kids, they call it a sports slump. All of a sudden, you're just not that good anymore.

SHAY: Yeah, I think that was it. But I still love being active. It's so much fun, especially when we do it together. As kids, Casey and I would go out and play basketball and we would go hard; we would work up that great competitive feeling. I'm finally experiencing that with you. You can throw and catch a football really well now, so we can go out and really play catch. It'll be fun once Gage and all of your other cousins start getting older and we can get into five-on-five basketball games out there. That's why I had five kids, after all—for a basketball team. I need a starting-five lineup!

It's so much fun being active, but there's a serious side to it, too. You've got to think that obesity, and all of its associated ailments, could be the thing that wipes out our species. Childhood obesity in particular is so important, because that is our next generation putting their lives on the line. When you think about common childhood diseases, you think about influenza, chicken pox, asthma. But at the top of the list these days is obesity, since more than a third of the children in the United States are overweight or obese, according to the Centers for Disease Control and Prevention.

Our obese kids are going to be the obese adults of the future, and they're going to carry all the baggage that goes with it: increased risk of diabetes, heart disease, stroke, bone and joint problems, and a bunch of cancers. Imagine all the other consequences of an over-weight population: just the other day, a group of retired generals in Kansas warned that people were getting "too fat to fight," and that over 70 percent of Kansans aged seventeen to twenty-four were unfit to serve in the military, many of them due to obesity. Health costs, too: an obese population is an unhealthy population, and even now, obesity-related illnesses cost a whopping $190 billion, according to the *Journal of Health Economics.* That's nearly 21 percent of annual medical spending in the United States. Fourteen billion dollars of that is down to childhood obesity.

So the problem is huge and immediate. Obesity is a different category of health problem in comparison to smoking, say. You only become a smoker when you start smoking. Eating is not an option. But if you go with the flow in today's world, eating processed food and drinking sodas and consuming larger portions, you will end up overweight or obese. Coasting is not an option for healthy living—not anymore.

One behavior I really do want to pass on to my kids is knowing how to shop for healthy food. It sucks that in our culture you can go to Jack in the Box and get ten pounds of food for four bucks, but there is a way to get healthy food for cheap.

You've got to be super alert when you go to the grocery store because sugar turns up where you least expect it—like in your orange juice, your bread, your salad dressings. But when you go into a supermarket to do your grocery shopping, I can tell you one secret that will lead you straight to the fresh, healthy, energy-giving food and help you bypass the processed sugar traps. You ready? Here it is.

- Stay on the perimeter. Don't even waste your time going to the middle of the grocery store. The whole, nutritious foods that the farmers bring to the supermarket, all that stuff is in the outer aisles. We do our shopping to the left of the entrance, where all the produce is, and to the far right, where the bread, whole grains, and nuts are. Along the back are the dairy and the eggs. Stay on the perimeter.
- Do not forget the universal rule about going to the grocery

store: never, never go hungry. Go after you've eaten, because if you go when you're hungry, you'll buy food that you don't need. You might want it, but you don't need it.

And for bonus points, here are two tips on buying food that is full of goodness:

- Iceberg lettuce is not lettuce. It is simply a transfer device for salad dressing. If it's white, there are hardly any nutrients in it. You want green—those nice dark green leaves, like romaine or baby spinach or kale. The greener, the better. Green is good.
- White bread is evil. Don't buy white bread. Buy whole grain; basically, any bread that has nuts, whole wheat, whole sesame seeds—any bread that's dark, that's what you want. That multigrain bread is a good source of fiber and protein, too. Make sure you go for one that has no high-fructose corn syrup.

Later this week, here's what Gavin and I are going to do: We're going to go to the store with two or three recipes in mind. We'll compare ingredients, weigh up organic versus non-organic, and look at the labels on salad dressing. I'm going to teach Gavin how to shop healthy. We'll be able to walk into the grocery store with ten dollars and get enough good, nutritious food to make a meal for ourselves and have plenty left over for the next day. How will we do that? We'll get our dark lettuce leaves, a pound of carrots for a buck—they have a ton of vitamins and carotene—and some of that great grainy bread we talked about. A pound bag of lentils, an onion, a cucumber, some salad dressing. The dressing is going to stretch your budget a little, especially if you choose something really nice, like a raspberry walnut dressing, but you have to have some salad dressing with your salad or it's just lame.

We'll make up a big batch of lentil soup that is so rich in protein and niacin and low in fat. To go with that, we'll make a nice healthy salad and some toast. Nothing's better than dipping your toast in some soup, you know what I'm saying?

You can get all of those ingredients for ten dollars. But let's have an honest moment here: when you look at your basket full of those goodies, it doesn't necessarily look fun. This doesn't look like a cheeseburger. This doesn't look like chicken tacos. But there are some real, whole foods that are healthy for you in there, and it's not a bad spread for ten dollars, right?

Feed your body with good, wholesome nutrients, and you'll feel the difference. Feed your kids the same thing and you'll be saving the human race.

Day 25

A Word to the Haters

WHILE WE'VE BEEN writing this book, a storm has erupted when people have seen the pre-release publicity. They're hating that we use the word "fat" in the title.

If you've read this far (that is, if you're not just flicking through the pages looking for cool pictures of my gorgeous wife) you'll know that Gavin and I have talked about the "f-word."

Would I say that my son is fat? No.

Would I say that I fear my son might develop the same unhealthy life patterns that I used to have and become fat—and more importantly, unhealthy? Yes.

I never want Gavin to be ashamed of who he is: a strong, caring, thoughtful human being. I do want to support him in every way to become healthier and find good foods and activities that will give him joy. That is what we are here for.

Seems that people are so ready to condemn others. It's something I've gained some experience in over these past few years on YouTube. Here are some of the things to hate about me:

- I buy water
- I drink water
- I run too much
- I eat raw foods
- I grow my beard
- I shave off my beard
- I gain too much weight
- I lose too much weight
- I go on a diet
- I fall off my diet

I've seen the comments. People say, *Oh Shay, you're so inconsistent.* Or *This is not the way you're supposed to do it.* Or *You're yo-yo dieting.*

Everyone is an expert, too. *My grandpa's aunt's boyfriend only ate meat for seven years and he lost 175 pounds, Shay. You should try that.* Or *You should try the all-shrimp diet, my best friend's neighbor's second cousin says that's the only one that works.* There are so many different ways to lose weight, but when it comes down to it, all you have to do is burn more calories than you consume. You can literally eat candy bars all day and lose weight. As long as you burn more calories than you eat, you're going to lose weight. You might not feel great, and you won't be healthy doing it that way, but what I'm saying is that you don't have to do it the way I'm doing it. Find your own way.

Many people are sincerely trying to be helpful, and that's different from the haters. You can't imagine the kind of things that I've read in the last nine years of my YouTube career. I'm pretty thick-skinned, and it never hurts my feelings; it's just water under the bridge. My mom gets caught up in it, though. She's my biggest fan, so when she sees people online saying mean things about me, she'll get on to the comments and fight with people. I tell her, "Mom, you've got to ignore it—they're just trolls."

I genuinely fear for the people who write hateful comments on my vlogs. I worry that their attitude is going to hurt them. My sole purpose in my ShayLoss videos is to motivate, encourage, and inspire people. The videos I make are intended to help people get past those hard things they've been avoiding for so long. If your first reaction is to say, "Shay's just lazy. He's all talk again," that doesn't hurt me. It hurts you. When you think you're putting your critique on to me, you're just projecting how you really feel inside. Maybe you're frustrated because you haven't been able to do the things I'm talking about, and you would dearly love to turn your own life around. Maybe you want to try to drag me down because misery loves company.

Do you remember Gavin talking about that kid at school who was being mean to another kid? And when Gavin stepped in, all he could think to say was, "Well, at least I'm not fat." That's the kid who grows up to post nasty comments on YouTube. He sees someone else doing the things he would do himself if he had the courage, and he lashes out. It says more about the pain inside than the person he's seeking to hurt.

At the end of each video, I'm gone. The haters are still there, living with themselves. Them, you, me—all of us have to live with ourselves. It's your life. It's your decision. It really doesn't matter what I say. What matters is how you answer when you ask yourself, *What am I going to do about my life?*

If your answer is, *I'm going to leave Shay a bad comment and tell him he's a fatso, that he gained his weight back and is a loser*, that won't help you. You trying to drag me down won't help you at all. Be selfish about it. Trying to hurt me only hurts you, so get selfish and take care of yourself.

I wouldn't say that criticism has had no effect on me, but the effect is that it has made me hypersensitive about being judgmental myself. Having been on the receiving end of it through YouTube for the past few years, I don't want to be that guy who tries to make himself feel like he's better than everyone else because everyone else is a jerk.

Most of the people who watch the vlogs and post comments don't have this problem, of course. It's just a few people out there. By far, the majority of emails, tweets, and comments we get are from people saying, *Thank you for letting us into your family's life and letting us see that it's possible to have a happy family.*

I love you. I'm going swimming now.

Day 26

Thirst Busters

SHAY: Life can feel pretty boring when you can't get that boost from sugar.

GAVIN: Like when you're on a plane and you want to get a Sprite.

SHAY: Right. I don't think we as a society realize how much we rely on sugar. How often we think, *Okay, now I get to have dessert*, or, *At least now I get to have my soda*. It gives you that dopamine kick, so when you can't have it, you're painfully reminded of it. Even though you don't realize you're searching for it every day, when it's gone, there's a big void. It can feel unfair, too. You might think to yourself, *We're going out to eat to celebrate. I want to have a good time, but I can't enjoy myself in the way that I'm used to.* Gavin, why do you think we eat?

GAVIN: To satisfy our hunger.

SHAY: So we can live, right? If we don't eat, we'll die. It's pretty fundamental stuff. But at the same time, food needs to be rewarding to
eat, or the human race would have died out not long after deciding that caves weren't the coolest places to live.

It takes a lot of effort to find and prepare food—these days it takes us
far less effort than it did for the Vikings, but even so, a lot of people
find food-gathering and preparation such a pain in the butt that they
would do anything to avoid it. Enter fast-food restaurants. I don't
think I would have done so well as a hunter-gatherer or a nomadic
berry-eater.

Even what we think of as the fundamental foods for "cooking from
scratch" have been through a bunch of processes before we pull them
off the grocery store's shelves. Our milk has been pasteurized, our
flour has been milled, our pasta is rolled and dried, ready to cook. We
don't make our own cheeses or harvest and grind our own herbs and
spices. We have it easy, when you think about it. If we were still in our
caves, finding a supply of high-calorie foods would be better than
winning the lottery. Sugar, fat, and salt were scarce, so finding a bee-
hive brimming with honey, or a nice, fatty caribou kidney would've
been a rare luxury.

How different things are for most of us today. Salt, sugar, and fat are
available on demand—even if you don't demand them, they're hidden
in so many of the food products we consume. We've reached a point
where we really do have too much of a good thing. On top of that, we've
turned eating into an event, which is both good and bad. I think it's a
wonderful thing to gather around the table as a family and enjoy one
another's company, but a lot of times, when we go out to a restaurant,

we're not even necessarily that hungry. We've probably consumed a decent number of calories already that day, so we're not eating to stay alive—we're eating to party. When you go out to eat, it's fun: the portions are lavish, and even the flavors seem bigger, especially when everything is deep-fried. Additives enhance the taste even more. Did you know there is a whole "flavor industry" in America that's worth $1.6 billion in revenues as of 2014? Industrially processed food is carefully crafted to maximize the qualities that make the food tastier: sweetness, saltiness, pleasing textures and colors—all the characteristics that make us want food. Scientists call it "food reward," and if you take a close look at what you eat every day, you'll most likely find plenty of those qualities. Seems like a no-brainer that we would choose to eat the things that are most appealing, but if you're trying to lose weight, those high-reward foods are a danger zone.

Think of your body as a finely tuned, highly expensive race car. You would take a lot of care about using the best high-octane gasoline and the right kind of oil to protect all the engine parts and give maximum performance, right? After all, it's going to mean the difference between standing on the winner's podium and coming in last. You would only put the best into that machine. How about treating your body like that? If you think about your body as a machine, you'll want to use it to do all the stuff you enjoy, function well, and have a long life.

This is where self-control comes in. You can still enjoy food while changing your focus from fun to fuel. Ask yourself, *Do I need this?* You know those times when you have eaten enough and you're full, but you eat those last three bites anyway because the food tastes so good? You've got to say no to that impulse. Anyway, the first few bites of a candy bar are the best part; after that, you're just eating it out of habit and because it's there. Each bite of food is less pleasant than the last, so the larger the portion, the less of a thrill you're getting by the time you're finished.

It's hard to pull self-control out of thin air, so you need to find new habits to replace the bad old ones. Habits don't just happen, they're made, so you can choose to form better habits. If you're a constant snacker, you might decide to rein that in a little by setting a timer that tells you when it's snack time. Before a meal, you might look at an old picture of yourself that shows how you want to look, or if you keep a food journal you might log what your previous meal was. Maybe you take a walk after dinner instead of having dessert. Exercise reduces brain responses to food reward, so that's going to have a double benefit for you.

New rewards will help lay those old habits to rest. You're looking for non-food-related treats here, something that makes you feel good. Set up a post-meal ritual, like phoning a buddy you haven't spoken to for a while, or shooting some hoops with your kids. Push ahead with a life goal: if you've always promised yourself that you will learn to speak Mandarin or play the guitar, set aside the time you would have been eating corn chips or brownies to do that.

Moderation matters, too. You can become maxed out by being too strict. You have to relax every once in a while, or you'll be wound too tight. You know that old saying, "All work and no play makes Jack a dull boy"? That Jack dude, he's always following the rules. You've got to let your hair down every once in a while. If you eat mostly fruits and vegetables, then steak and ice cream every once in a while will not only *not* hurt you, they'll feel like a celebration.

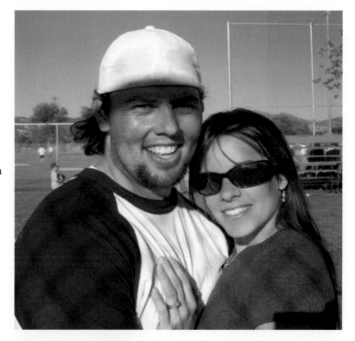

Me and Colette in 2006, right before my fast pitch softball game.

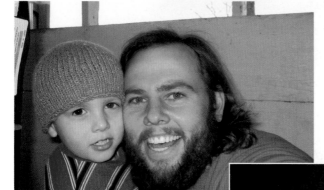

Me and Gavin on our father-son ski trip to Pebble Creek in 2007.

Gavin eating a cookie at the Pebble Creek ski lodge.

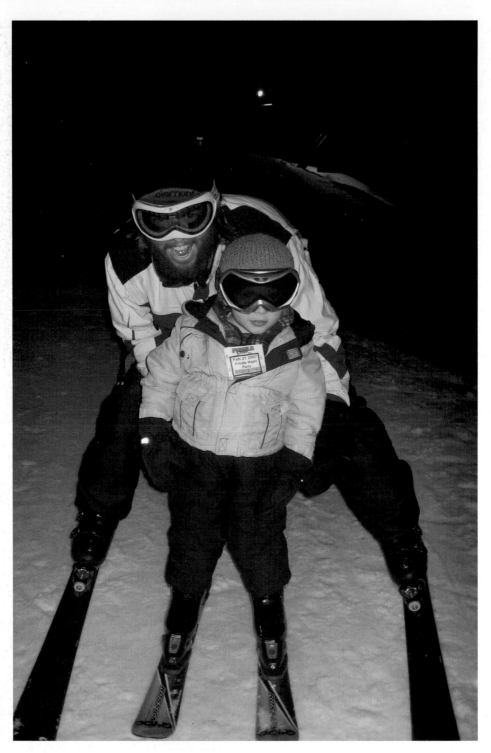

Gavin's first time on skis! He switched to snowboarding right after.

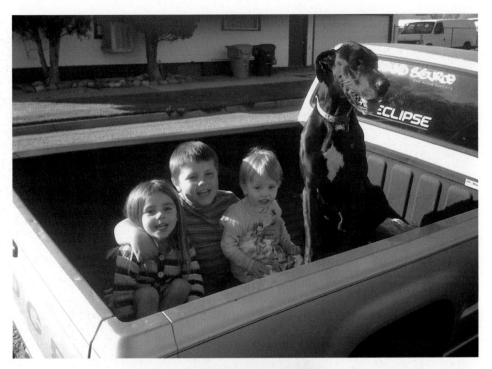

ABOVE: Our first four kids! Gavin, Avia, Emmi, and our family dog, Malachi. I drove this blue Dodge sixty miles round-trip every weekday to host the Z103 night show from six p.m. to midnight for a paycheck of $8.50 an hour.

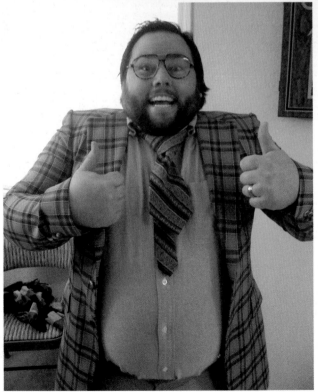

LEFT: Early attempt at a Chris Farley impression.

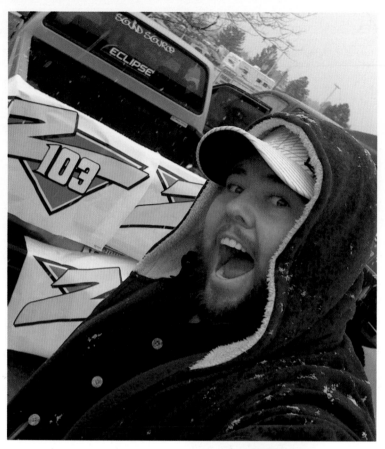

ABOVE: In the parking lot of the local post office in Pocatello, Idaho, for a live radio remote broadcast for Z103.

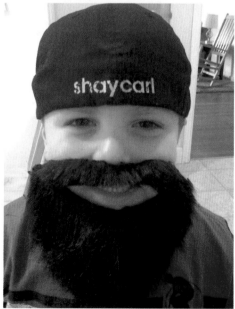

Like father, like son. Gavin wearing a fake beard and the first run of Shaycarl hats in 2008.

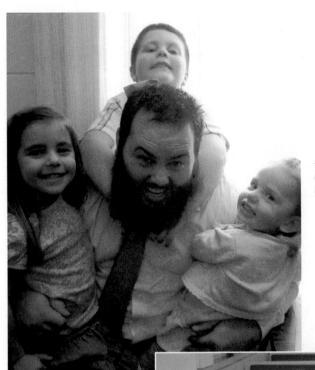

At church with Gavin, Avia, and Emmi. Also pictured: Glorious Shaybeard #1.

Avia, Emmi, and Gavin eating chicken nuggets at McDonald's.

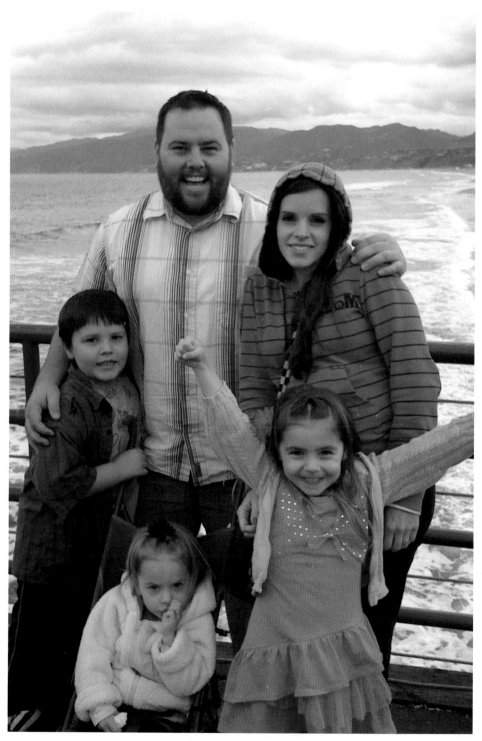

The Shaytards at the Santa Monica Pier in 2009, right after we moved to LA.

Outside of the famous El Capitan Theatre in Hollywood, right after we moved to LA.

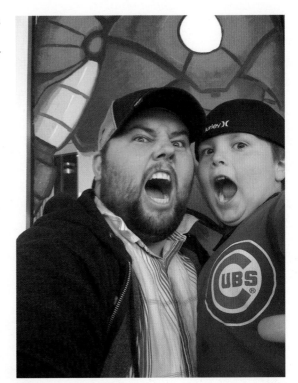

BELOW: Me, Avia, Emmi, and Gavin in 2009 after shooting the "WE FOUND IT" video for my Shaycarl channel on YouTube.

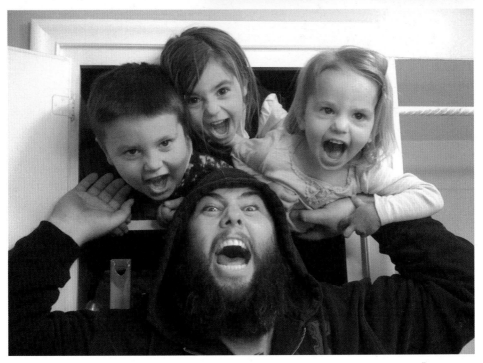

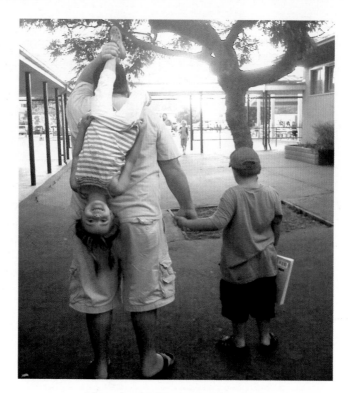

After school in Venice Beach in 2009.

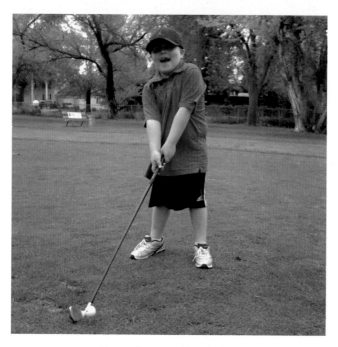

Gavin playing golf with dad!

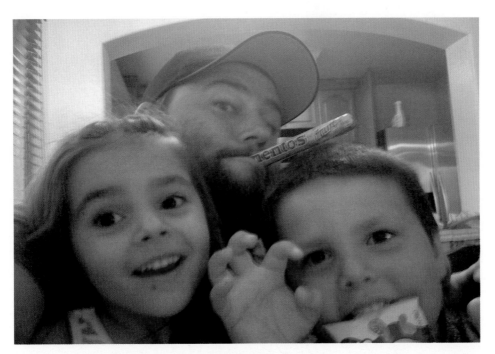

Our second house in LA was half a block away from a corner market, where it was really easy to pick up a "treat."

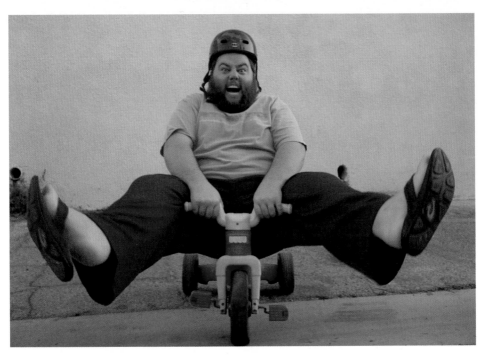

Me on a tricycle in 2009, not exactly at the peak of health and fitness. #terrifying

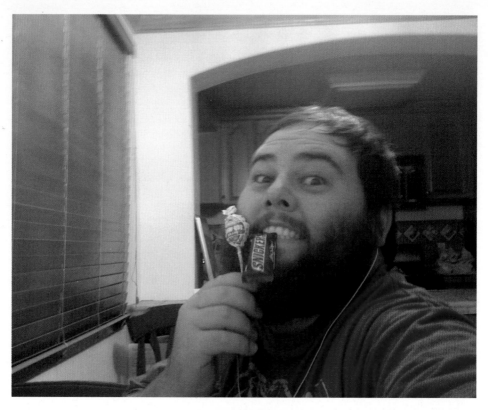

More candy! More beard!

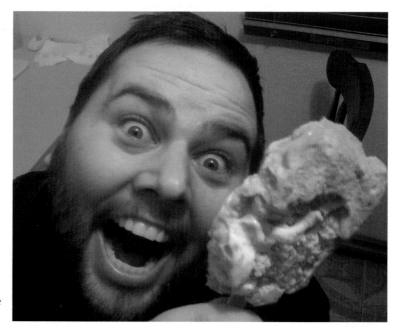

Fat guys eat ice cream in all forms. Here, we see it on a stick.

First juice to kick off my twenty-day raw food cleanse in 2009.

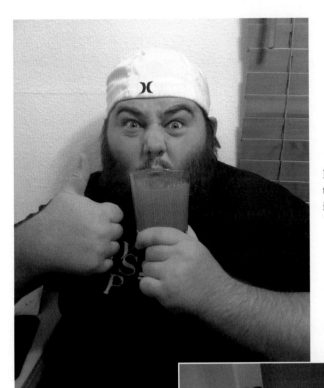

I lost twenty pounds in twenty days during my raw food cleanse, which ended on Thanksgiving Day in 2009. This was the first real food I got to eat. I think I ate half of this turkey!

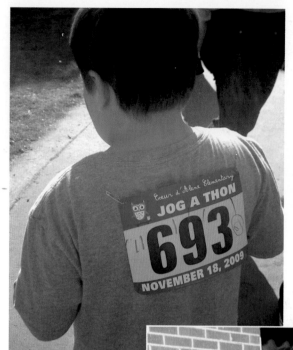

Gavin's kindergarten Jog-A-Thon in Venice Beach in November 2009.

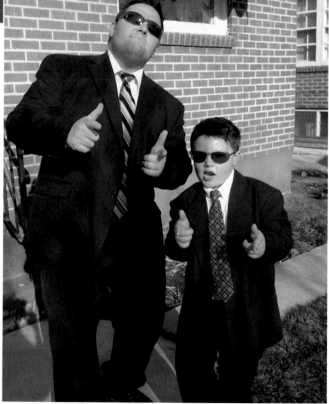

Two rad dudes pointing our fingers at the camera before church.

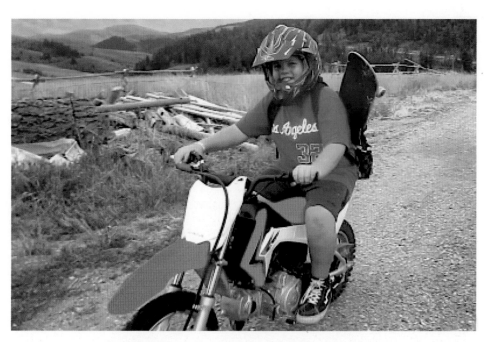

Gavin riding a motorcycle with a skateboard strapped to his back in the mountains of Idaho in 2014.

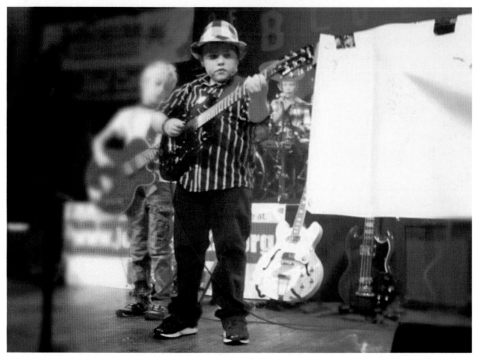

Gavin playing electric guitar onstage at the House of Blues in Hollywood.

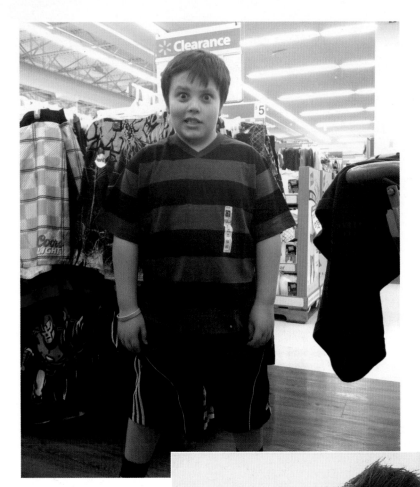

ABOVE: Shopping for school clothes with Gavin at Walmart.

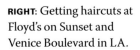

RIGHT: Getting haircuts at Floyd's on Sunset and Venice Boulevard in LA.

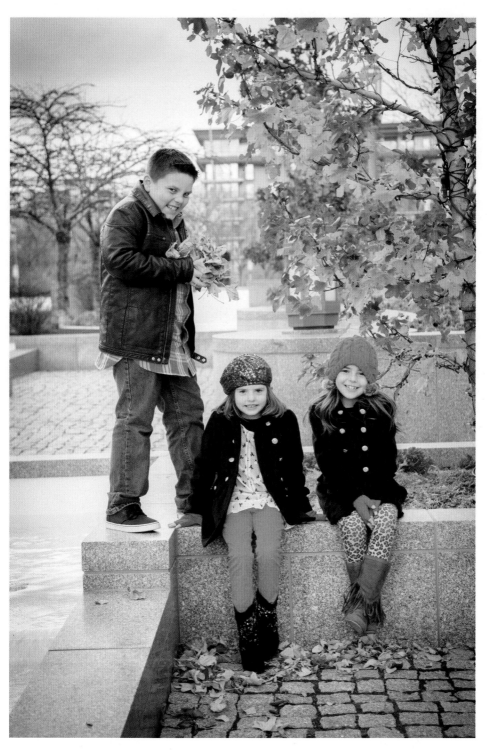

The Shaytards Christmas calendar photo shoot at Salt Lake City in November 2014.

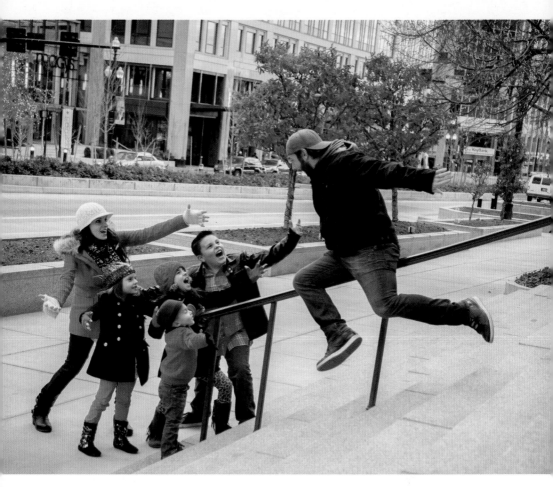

<3

You know, my mom did it hard when she was growing up. She didn't have a great deal of money in her family. After she and Dad married, Dad studied online with DeVry University and got his electrical engineering qualifications. So when we finally had some money, my mom wanted to celebrate. Because we're Latter-day Saints, we don't drink, so she splurged the only way she knew how: we'd go out to Circle K for hot dogs and those mega fountain drinks, or we'd get a treat at the gas station, where it's all Laffy Taffy and Slurpees and Coke and Skittles. Every time we went on a road trip, we'd stop to get gas and load up on giant Cokes and sunflower seeds and licorice. It's a rush and it's fun, but you just end up with a belly full of sugar and chemicals.

I remember one time when my mom picked us up from school for lunch as a surprise. I was about nine years old and my brother, Casey, was seven. She had left work early to treat us to a lunch of nachos and Thirst Busters at the nearest Circle K. It was 1989, and the very biggest fountain drink they had was thirty-two ounces. I remember it looked HUGE. But my mom always wanted us to have the best and biggest, so we both got thirty-two-ounce Thirst Busters. It came in a bright orange cup that had blue 3-D lettering on the side that said, in all caps, THIRST BUSTERS. It looked *awesome*.

My mom dropped us off back at school, and Casey and I strode onto campus with our giant cups. I vividly remember that two sixth graders were sitting on some stairs, and as we walked by, one of them said, "Whoooa! Thirty-two ouncers?!" The way he said it made me feel cool and grown-up, like he was impressed that I was the kind of person who could handle a thirty-two-ouncer.

Can you imagine what that moment was like for a nine-year-old kid? That definitely put some swagger in my step. *Yeah, that's right, I might only be a kid, but I'm bursting thirst like a big boy!* I carried that cup around like a badge of honor; for me, it was the equivalent of walking around with a T-shirt that advertised my bench press max on it. It didn't matter that I had to use both of my very small nine-year-old hands to carry my soda trophy back to my second-grade classroom; I felt like a champ.

Since then, I've come to realize that being able to eat and drink a lot isn't really a badge of honor, even if it *does* impress some people along the way. One of the best ways to honor yourself is to respect your body. I think what makes me nostalgic about that memory isn't the taste of Thirst Busters, but what it represents for me: quality time with my mom. When you're used to positively associating junk food with good memories and feelings, take a minute to understand the underlying feeling. That's what you should carry forward with you. Leave the Thirst Busters behind. Trust me, that's not the part you'll miss when all is said and done.

Day 27

Secrets in Plain Sight

I'VE BEEN THINKING AGAIN about my epic bike ride to Malibu, that time when I just started riding my bike and went farther each day until I found the end of the bike path. Around that time people were mentioning in the vlogs that I was looking healthy. *Dang, Shay, you're really looking skinny, you're doing a good job.*

After my triumphant discovery of the end of the Malibu bike path, I was riding back home and thinking how awesome it was that what I was doing was finally working. As a YouTuber, I want to share these things with my audience to motivate them, too, so I started to think about what I had been doing to lose weight and get healthy. What exactly had I done that had made a difference? *Okay, I've been exercising every day. I'm eating healthy. I'm drinking a lot of water. I'm working hard. I'm not giving up.* But the YouTuber part of my mind stopped that line of thought in its tracks. *Hang on, I can't say that to my audience because they're just going to stop me and say, Aw Shay, that's just a cliché.*

I could already feel the negative feedback that would come from me saying this is how I did it. I needed some other secret way, a mysterious ingredient or a special technique. But then as I pedaled along, debating it in my mind, I came to the conclusion that this *is* what I've been doing, this *is* how I've lost weight. Those were the answers to how I had lost thirty pounds; this was why I felt great and had more energy—and how I made it to the end of that bike path. That's all it was. It's about not quitting, working hard, going for my bike ride every day, eating healthy, and drinking water. No matter how many people write in the comments, *Well that's just a cliché*, those are my secrets to a healthier life.

A phrase came to me and hit me so hard that I had to pull my bike over and tweet it. It's a saying I've started to live my life by, and it is this: the secrets to life are hidden behind the word "cliché."

The things that we call clichés are the things we need to perk up and listen to. Those clichés should become our mantras, the principles that drive our everyday actions. Anything you hear that's a cliché, most people gloss over it. "That's the obvious answer," they say, and they keep looking for something more obscure and less obvious. But those are the secrets. They're so obvious and ingrained in our culture and our stories. Sometimes they're embedded in the stories we tell our kids, like *The Little Engine That Could*: "I think I can, I think I can." Morals about not giving up and working hard are the secret to success.

I've switched my thinking now, so every time I hear something that sounds like a cheesy motivational quote, or something too obvious, instead of glossing over it or ignoring it, I've trained my ears to perk up and listen. Most people respond with *Yeah, yeah, I've heard this a million times.* Anytime I hear something like that, I figure truth is being spoken in that moment. Instead of deriding it, we should revere it, because that's how you get to happy, that's how you become successful: by doing these things that we all know, but for some reason, we all just ignore.

So there you go. Those are the secrets to life: working hard, not quitting, exercise—all the commonsense things. After I lost a hundred pounds, so many people I met would ask me, "How did you do it? How can I do it?" Once a guy asked me that in church, and I answered him, "I worked my ass off." Woah, I was in church, I shouldn't have been swearing—but that's what I said because that was the truth. "There is no secret," I told him. I ate fruits and vegetables, drank water, and ran, so I lost weight. It's simple—hard sometimes, for sure, but simple. That's how you do it.

It sucks doing the hard things. But if you get down to brass tacks, that's what it's about. It's about doing the things you don't want to do because they're hard. It's easier to sit on the couch. It's easier to eat food that's delicious. It's easier to sleep in. It's easier to procrastinate and not do your homework and not make your bed and not clean your room. It's easier to stuff all the junk under your bed and not organize it, and shove things in your closet or in the trunk of your car.

But what I'm finding is, it's easier to truly relax when you have done the hard things throughout the day. There's an old saying, and I'm going to butcher it, but it goes something like, "Laziness is the hardest job of all, because you can never rest from it."

This is tough talk right now, people. I want to do the hard things, because that is what successful people do. Successful people make it a habit to do the things that you don't want to do, like making your bed, doing your homework, flossing and brushing your teeth, exercising, eating healthy, and drinking plenty of water. The things that suck to do. Replying to emails—I'm really bad at that. Successful people have made it a habit of doing the hard things.

So for this one month, I've been asking myself with every decision that I make, at every crossroads, "What is the hard way?"

Did you ever grow up with somebody successful who always stuck to the books and did what they were supposed to do? Did you maybe say to yourself, *Oh, look at Mr. Goody Two Shoes*. People sneer at that, but those people who do what they're supposed to do, they have success because they've made a habit to do the hard things.

I feel like I'm a pretty successful guy and I get some stuff done, but I know I could do way better. I know I could turn the computer off and go to bed earlier, I know I could wake up earlier, I know I could reply to emails. There are projects and opportunities that I want to do. There're two new projects that I know I could get started. I'm not going to tell you what they are, but I've been procrastinating over them for the past six months because they require extra work that I don't want to do.

I just want to do my daily vlogs and then play with my kids and eat dinner and watch TV with my wife and go to bed, and then wake up around nine. But I know that I can live better. I know that I can do more. So for these thirty days, I want to live in a way so that every time I'm about to make a decision about how I'm going to live my life, I immediately think, *What's the hard thing?* It's not enough to do the bare minimum—I want to challenge myself in every way, beyond the healthy living that we've been talking about here.

A lot of you guys post comments that say things like, *Oh Shay, you're so lucky. You've got all this money from YouTube now.* The reason that I have all these things, a beautiful wife, and this amazing house is because I've chosen that life. That's what I wanted for myself. That's what I've always wanted. Ever since I was a kid growing up, I've always looked up to people who were successful and who worked hard and achieved things. When I was growing up, I knew this family where the dad was a dentist and they had more money than everybody else. Everybody hated them because they had a boat and they got to go to Hawaii on holidays. But I used to wonder, *Why don't you like those people? Doesn't everybody want to be successful, have nice things, and live the good life?* Instead of complaining and being jealous of those people, why not say, *I want to be like that guy, so I'm going to do what he does. I want to be rich, too.* Who doesn't, right? Who doesn't want the nice things? You can have them by doing what rich people do.

If you want to be fat, do what a fat person does. If you want to be skinny, do what a skinny person does. It's as simple as that. Just by making those choices and changing your life, it's possible. I know you can do it. I know you can. You've just got to make that choice. It's a mighty change of heart that you have to have within yourself. You have to get sick and tired of being sick and tired.

It's about being vigilant in your life. You're being vigilant about your body, about the everyday choices you make. I believe that you're either slowly getting better every day, or you're slowly getting worse every day. If you're not actively engaging in an effort to increase your success, then you're going to tilt downward and you're going to slowly go down.

A lot of you ask me for weight loss-tips and what they should do. There's no secret, people. You pick any friggin' diet plan out there. Any plan. You go on the Internet and type in "Diet plan" or "How to lose weight." Anything that comes up—pick it and do it. If you do it, you will succeed. I guarantee. Doesn't matter what it is, as long as you do it. That's the secret: action. The doing is what makes things move.

If you really want to lose weight, you can't just tinker around the edges of your life, cut out a few carbs or walk around the block once a week. You've got to work hard. Nothing comes without working. Everything happens because of you doing something. Nothing is ever going to happen without action. Work will work when nothing else will work.

Day 28

Health *Hurts*!

TODAY WAS NOT a good running day for me. I laced up my shoes and put my headphones on and went out there, but pretty much from the time I started, I wanted to go back so bad. Every step my head was saying, *Stop, just stop.* My ankle was hurting me, and I just wanted to be back in my bed. It was one of those mornings, but I told myself, *No—listen to some music, think about something else, you're not stopping.* For a mile I was hating it every step of the way. Inside my head, the argument kept going on: *Shay, this is your mind speaking and I'm in charge. I'm running the ship right now and you are going to do this.* Meanwhile, the other part of my head was saying, *This is stupid, why am I doing this?*

After a mile something happened: everything loosened up, I got a sweat going, and this song hit on shuffle. You know how you can get the perfect song at the perfect time? Maybe a nice breeze comes along and you get a really good inhale of oxygen and you find your second wind—although I hadn't even gotten my first wind at that point because I was hating it so badly. Anyway, I locked in on that song and suddenly my ankle felt better. This song was jamming and I started running faster and I saw a lady jogging who looked like she was in pretty good shape and I passed her, and boom—I was in the zone. The next four songs made it seem as if my iPod just knew what I needed to hear, and I went four miles. It felt amazing. I started using my arms and listening to my heartbeat, and I could feel my whole body was like a machine. It felt so good to work it.

You know what's exciting? Right now I feel like I'm in that optimal growth zone, where I'm able to do more than I could a week ago or a month ago. A lot of people write in and say, *Shay, I could never do a marathon.* Yes you can. The secret is just pushing yourself a little farther than you stopped last time. If you can only walk around your block once, the next day try to do it twice. That's all it is: building on it little by little over time. You have to be in charge, too, to able to say, "No, body, I am in control up here. I am in charge, and I say you're going to do this because I know it's good for you." When you push on through, by the end of your walk or run you're going to be feeling good and you'll be motivated to do it again.

Earlier this week I was driving in my truck on Venice Boulevard, right next to Venice High School, where they shot the outdoor scenes for *Grease.* I was waiting at a stoplight next to a Los Angeles public transport bus, and I looked up at the driver. This dude looked like me: he was probably thirty-five or forty years old with a beard, balding, but he weighed around three hundred pounds, or maybe a bit more.

As I looked at this guy on the bus, I could tell that his seat belt was really tight on him, cutting through his gut with fat spilling out on each side.

I remembered exactly how that felt: I'd been on many airplanes where I had to extend the seatbelt clip all the way out to its maximum length just so I could clip it on. I'd been the fat guy they have to squeeze on to the rides at Disneyland. I know what it's like to suck in as much as you can so that you can go on the rides with your kids. I sat there looking at this bus driver, and I knew how horrible that felt, how claustrophobic, how debilitating and depressing. A lot of times the only way you overcome that depression is with the excitement of the next meal. I had felt that way for so long, and I was so glad that I don't feel that way anymore.

I knew that it only took me six months to not feel that way, and as I looked at that guy sitting on that bus, constrained by that seat belt, I knew in my head that if he would just commit to six months of serious diet change and exercise, he would feel amazing, like me. Six months is such a short time! How many Christmases have gone by in the blink of an eye—five Christmases, ten Christmases, they just fly by. How long has it been since that school reunion when you felt embarrassed by how big you've gotten? Six months is nothing.

I'm making it sound easy, but I know it's not. As humans, we tend to want what's easy. We're always trying to avoid pain. Almost all of the choices we make are based on that one thing: avoiding pain. Maybe exercise doesn't hurt, strictly speaking, but it's uncomfortable. In relative terms, it's more painful than lying on the couch.

I love this quote from Tony Robbins: "Change happens when the pain of staying the same is greater than the pain of change." What that means for me is that it is more painful for me to stay as I am—not being able to sleep very well, not being able to run around with my kids without getting winded, feeling like crap, having my pants be too tight on my waist, going out in public and feeling that everyone is staring at me because I'm fat. That pain is greater than the pain of exercising and eating healthy and not being able to have my Coca-Cola Classic. That is when change happens: when it's easier to do even the things you don't necessarily want to do than to experience the pain of being fat and feeling like crap.

Once you make that decision to change, there are some things you can do to reduce the pain. As you know, years ago I had a job making and installing granite countertops. When I was working at the granite shop, I would sit and watch the clock. I hated being there, and I hated those two hands that were stuck inside that circle on the wall, because they were in charge of me. When that hand got to this number and the other hand reached that other number, then I could go be myself, be with my family, and do what I wanted to do. Until then, I had to be there in that shop.

It felt like indentured servitude. You clock-in each morning with a card with your number on it, and you put it in a machine that makes a little clunking sound that really means, *You're ours now!* Then for the rest of the day you stare at the clock while you're doing the thing they tell you to do so that they'll trade you this amount of money for this amount of time. Your life is exchanged for money by the hour. I'd get out of work at five o'clock, so at four thirty, when I had thirty minutes left, I'd be dying. The voice in my head would be saying, *It's 4:31. Now it's 4:32.* We've all done that at some point, right? I did it in school, too—I used to stare at that dang hand and it just wouldn't move. It was always stuck right there, about a quarter turn from where you wanted it to be.

One day I was staring at the clock in the granite shop. It was four thirty, and I had a half hour left, and man, I was dreading that last half hour. You know that feeling when you're avoiding doing anything because you're about to leave? It's that panicky feeling that maybe you should hide from the boss and get under the desk so you can just leave when that last thirty minutes is up. I hated that feeling. It was annoying to feel that way, so I decided I was just going to clean the shop.

The shop was a mess: there was a pile of silicone bottles in one corner and stacks of old granite fragments along the other wall. So I just started working away there, trying to make my work area better. I figured that it would be so nice if I could get all this crap out of the way and I could put my stereo there. I get cleaning and working and I looked up at the clock and it was five thirty. I couldn't believe it; I had stayed past the time when I could have left work. Colette had been texting me but I had just lost myself in the work. Those thirty minutes that drag on for an eternity had turned into an hour, and yet it felt like just five seconds had passed.

Because I changed the way I was looking at the situation, my paradigm, if you like to call it that, shifted. Now, I wasn't truly enslaved, but people who have been in jail or in prison camps use this kind of mentality to survive. In their minds they say, *None of this matters. I can choose to be happy. I can sing inside my head. I can think of a poem, or a great experience that I've had. No one can take that away from me, that's still mine.*

No matter what situation you're in, however tedious or horrible or devastating, you can still be happy. You can go into that place where nothing that's happening—the dreary school day, the teacher shouting, the granite shop, the clock, prison—none of that can get to you if you're free inside your mind. You always control that space.

It's true for me and it's true for Gavin. In any situation where you're thinking, *This sucks, I'm riding up this hill on my bicycle and I'm dying. Why is Dad going so fast?* You don't have to think those thoughts. Instead, you could think, *It's summer and I'm writing a book. I'm going to play football with my cousins later. I'm going to be in sixth grade next year.* There are so many good things that are happening, and once you get into that mentality, your whole mind-set changes. You get into the motivation cycle that we talked about earlier: you start the wheels rolling, then you see some results, so you get inspired and you have more successes and you work harder. It's the same with healthy living, weight loss, and getting over the procrastination. You see the results of your efforts and the wheels start turning over and over and you just . . . go.

Day 29

Tiny Robots

This morning we talked about how if they invented little robots that made you physically stronger and healthier but you didn't have to do anything, would you use them. And I say no because I want to do the work myself. I don't want some tiny robot doing it for me.

The future is going to be an amazing place to be. We're on the cusp of being able to replace body parts that malfunction and being able to embed data into our bodies, a future where death itself is optional.

Even now, surgeons have worked out how to implant a tiny telescope in the eye, which helps give back the vision that is lost through macular degeneration, which is a huge cause of blindness for older people. There's some amazing research in regenerating damaged tissues and organs by injecting stem cells or implanting organs that have been bioengineered in a lab from stem cells that were harvested from the patient, so there's less risk the body will reject them. They've already tried it out with a bunch of different tissues and organs: skin, blood vessels, knee cartilage, windpipes, even bladders.

Three-dimensional printing is another thing scientists are experimenting with to build body parts. Instead of ink, they use cells to print ear lobes and noses and skin.

We're going to go way beyond Google Glass. There will be a time when Gavin will wake up to see three emails (or whatever the future equivalent of an email is) from me, all embedded in front of his eyes in a contact lens that contains all of his data, and he can read them just by deciding to. Or he'll hit delete by thinking it . . . but he better reply to his dad with his eyeball computer, or he's grounded!

This is all massively exciting, but it all raises huge ethical issues. How much of your body can you replace before you are no longer strictly human? Right now, I don't think too many people would dispute that technology that replaces a missing limb or restores sight doesn't make anyone less human. But what about if technology could boost your brain into a supercomputer? When do doctors move from healing to playing God? If you know that you can just hand over your credit card and pick up a new lung from a laboratory, does that make it okay to smoke a pack of cigarettes a day? Will the rich get healthier while the poor get sicker just because wealthy people can afford to pay for replacement hearts or livers? And if you could download your brain to a computer chip and implant it in another body when your own body wears out, would you do it?

You know by now that I'm a big believer in doing the work, that sometimes our goals for a healthy body can only be achieved by working hard and doing the things that don't come so easily. Somewhere in the future, though, your doctor might simply prescribe a fat-burning pill. That may not be too far in the future, either: the Harvard Stem Cell Institute has found a way to trick the body's white fat cells into thinking they're brown, so they behave like brown fat cells by burning excess energy instead of storing it around our bodies.

Think about that. If there was a pill you could swallow or a computer that could activate your body to make you leaner and fitter without having to run or lift weights or swim or ride a bike, would you take it?

GAVIN: In my opinion, I don't want someone to make me thinner. I want to do it myself.

SHAY: You don't want a computer to do it?

GAVIN: No, I want to do the work myself.

SHAY: I didn't think about it like that. I was thinking maybe it would be cool, but straight away, you're saying, "I want to work for it." I wish I'd said that!

Thinking about that "magic pill"—it's like when you see someone who has achieved something that you would like to achieve for yourself—success in their work life, say—and you think, *Oh yeah, that's where I want to be, too.* But if I had what they had without earning it, there's no honor in that. We are on this Earth to learn, and the only way to learn is through experience—which is another way of saying the only way to learn is by doing the work.

The sooner you can accept that in life you have to work hard, the happier you will be. There will always be problems that you will have to overcome. But there is happiness to be achieved by saying, *That's just part of life, and I'm going to do the work every day with a smile on my face.*

People ask me about the future of YouTube and where I think I will be in five years' time. It's a giant train I'm riding; I don't know where it's going to go and how long the journey will take, but I'm just riding it as long and as fast as I can. The industry is gaining legitimacy every day, and the more that happens, the longer I foresee it going. Barring some crazy disaster, I can see it evolving the way it has the past four years, just growing exponentially faster and faster and bigger and bigger. We'll just adapt and grow with it. The sky's the limit.

I know for a fact there are some really cool opportunities ahead—not just for me, but for everybody. There's a real feeling of abundance; it just takes time for the cool things to come together. We've got to work at it and put the time in, and eventually we'll see the fruits of our labor. My goal is that I always want to be in control of what I'm doing, creating things that I like and that other people will like as well. If I can just keep doing that and keep being able to make a living, to provide for my family and pay those stupid bills that keep turning up, I'll keep doing the exact same things but at a different level. I love that with YouTube, I can wake up tomorrow and say, *I want to make a music video about gorillas in unitards*; think of a crazy idea, put it together, and present it for people to watch. I just want to keep doing that.

As far as the technology goes, as Apple TV and Google TV become more mainstream, they're going to take the Internet viewing experience to television. That will offer people what they are used to, which is sitting on their couch and watching things that entertain and inform them. There will be a fusion of YouTube and the TV scene—but that's not to say that I want to be making TV shows. I like where we're at now. I would stay right on my Shaytards and Shaycarl channels for the rest of time, because I don't ever want to lose the freedom I have to create the things I enjoy. I want to keep working on this platform that we have built and making it stronger. Empowering it. I want to be like William Wallace, leading the troops into the battlefield of entertainment!

When I think about the future, I also think about my children being all grown up. Listening to Gavin talk today about not wanting tiny robots doing the work makes me feel like he really is going to be a remarkable young man and appreciate the value of work. He won't be afraid of taking the harder path.

The future is looking brighter by the day.

Day 30

We Did It!

THIRTY DAYS—ARE YOU SERIOUS? We hit thirty days! Gavin, where did Mom hide the candy? I'm off to the ice-cream store now. See ya!

Kidding. Just kidding. But I honestly did get to a point where I wasn't even counting the days. We've just gotten used to living this way, and we've learned how to cope with it. It's definitely way easier now than it was in the beginning, so I'm not thinking, *When can I have sugar again?* Colette is more that way than I am; she's been saying, "Hey, when you can have sugar again, can we go out for ice cream?" She has plans for us, and now we can tell her, this weekend, we can do them.

Gavin and me working together has been such a great experience. We've been really physical, doing a lot of activities. I've been proud of Gavin and he's looking and feeling so good. He's been working hard, walking and running those hills. We went to CrossFit together the other morning, and he was definitely kicking butt. I think he's on the right path, and we're not going to stop.

SHAY: Gavin, have you weighed yourself at all since that last time?

GAVIN: Yeah, I'm still my same weight. One hundred and fifty-four pounds.

SHAY: What were you before we started?

GAVIN: One hundred and sixty-one.

SHAY: Well, that's cool—seven pounds is a lot, you wouldn't want to lose more than that in a month. Best of all, I love that you just said your weight without seeming ashamed, and that was something that I think was hard for you before. And I don't think either of us has slipped up or cheated, have we?

GAVIN: Well, okay, there were a couple of times when you thought I was cheating.

SHAY: You snapped at me the other day for accusing you of cheating, even though I knew you hadn't. You were feeding something to Daxton—what was it?

GAVIN: A cupcake.

SHAY: Oh yeah, we were at my mom's house and she had made cup-cakes, and you walked into the room with cupcake crumbs all over yourself. I said, "Gavin, what's that?" And you told me, "I didn't eat any!" Then Daxton comes walking in and he has cup-cake all over his face, so I could tell you were just being a good big brother and helping the little guy with a cupcake. Were you tempted to have a few crumbs too?

GAVIN: No. Well, just the frosting on my fingers. I did want to lick that off.

You know, over the past few years, I've done a bunch of different challenges—no candy or pop for a year, raw food diets, training for a marathon—and every single one of them has made me healthier and more aware of how I use my body and what I put into it. But none of them has had such a deep impact as this challenge Gavin and I have just finished here. This has done more than change my body; it has changed my heart. I've come to see my son in a new way, gained a deeper appreciation for his strengths, and been so encouraged by having him alongside me every step of the way.

I started this thing wanting to pass on to Gavin some of the things I've learned about living a healthy life. I believe it has worked, too, because I see the differences in him; he's getting faster and more agile, and he looks leaner and fitter. Since the challenge, we've talked about how good we feel, and we're both committed to making this an enduring part of our lives, not just a blip on the screen.

As you've read alongside us about our struggles and successes over these last thirty days, I hope it's made you start to think about asking your own son, daughter, mom, dad, cousin, neighbor, best friend—whoever it might be—to team up with you to create positive change in your own lives. Maybe you'll do a thirty-day challenge like us, or maybe you'll pick some other lifestyle change that's just right for you. One thing you will definitely discover is that, together, we're stronger than we could ever imagine.

Time and pressure, my friends. Time and pressure. Just keeping pushing on.

I love you guys. Be well.

Acknowledgments

AS WE LOOK BACK on the pathway of our lives that have led each of us to this very moment in time, we often—if not always—see powerful people who seem purposely perched and prepared to propel us past potential pessimistic pot holes; honest men and women who, for some reason, have given their unconditional love in the absence of any hope for payment or acclaim. Most of these people are usually taken for granted until they die, unless you get the opportunity to write about them in the acknowledgments of your book . . . so NOW is the time for some major shout-outs!

First and foremost, I want to give major props to my son, Gavin Butler, for his bravery in talking about his feelings and standing up to the bullies of the world. He is wise beyond his years and one of my best friends.

To my parents, Carl and Laurie Butler! They have guided me, prepared me, and supported me through every single second of my life. They gave me my sense of humor and taught me how to work and laugh. Without them there would be one less beard in the world, and that is a horrible thing to imagine.

To my friend, Amy Finnerty, and the team at Maker Studios who watch my back in the boardrooms of the social media world.

To my editor, Jhanteigh Kupihea, for her eternal patience and clear eyes amongst a hailstorm of "shay ideas."

To my very favorite person from the country of Australia, Sally Collings, who came in after I had written three chapters in seven months and took the reins and crossed the t's and dotted the i's and asked the good questions that needed to be asked without ever getting in the way.

Lastly, to my very best friend and eternal companion Colette. I loved you the very first day I saw you, and ever after.

About the Author

SHAY BUTLER IS an award-winning digital entrepreneur and vlogger. His YouTube channels attract millions of subscribers, and he has been hailed as one of the "most successful video entrepreneurs on YouTube" by Forbes.com. Butler is a cofounding talent of Maker Studios. He lives in Idaho with his wife, Colette, and five children. **GAVIN BUTLER** is his eldest son.